The Simplicity of Dementia

The Simplicity of Dementia
A Guide for Family and Carers

Huub Buijssen

Jessica Kingsley Publishers
London and Philadelphia

The right of Huub Buijssen to be identified as author of this work has been asserted by him in accordance with the Copyright, Designs and Patents Act 1988.

First published in Dutch in 1999 by De Stiel, Nijmegen and Tred Uitgeverij, Tilburg as *De heldere eenvoud van dementie: Een gids voor dee familie.*

First published in English in 2005
by Jessica Kingsley Publishers
116 Pentonville Road
London N1 9JB, UK
and
400 Market Street, Suite 400
Philadelphia, PA 19106, USA
www.jkp.com

Copyright © Huub Buijssen 2005
Second impression 2005

Library of Congress Cataloging in Publication Data
Buijssen, H. P. J.
[Heldere eenvoud van dementie. English]
The simplicity of dementia : a guide for family and carers / Huub Buijssen.
p. cm.
Includes bibliographical references and index.
ISBN-13: 978-1-84310-321-9 (pbk.)
ISBN-10: 1-84310-321-4 (pbk.)
1. Dementia. 2. Caregivers. 3. Dementia--Patients--Care. 4. Dementia--Patients--Family relationships. I. Title.
RC521.B856 2005
616.8'3--dc22

2004027024

British Library Cataloguing in Publication Data
A CIP catalogue record for this book is available from the British Library

ISBN-13: 978 1 84310 321 9
ISBN-10: 1 84310 321 4

Printed and Bound in Great Britain by
Athenaeum Press, Gateshead, Tyne and Wear

For my mother,
who gave her all to keep Father at home
for as long as was conceivably possible

The author would like to thank the publishers and authors who have kindly given permission to reproduce the following material:

Quotes on pp.13, 57, 144, 161–2 and 168–9 from *Ze is de vioolmuziek vergeten* (1995) by Marjan van den Berg, published by Van Reemst. Used with permission from the author.

Quotes on pp.18, 42, 58 and 65 from *We komen niet meer waar we geweest zijn* (1993) by Ingrid H. van Delft, published by Anthos. Used with permission from the author.

Quotes on pp.26–7 and 93–4 from *Remind me who I am again* (1998) by Linda Grant, published by Granta Books. Used with permission from A.P. Watt Ltd on behalf of Linda Grant.

Quote on p.32 from *Memory* (1987) by Margaret Mahy, published by Collins Flamingo. Used with permission from HarperCollins Publishers Ltd and Watson Little.

Quote on p.35 from *De moeder van Nicolien* (1999) by J.J. Voskuil, published by G.A. van Oorschot. Used with permission from the publisher.

Quotes on pp.38–9, 67–8, 78–9, 81 and 147–8 from *Dubbel verlies* (1997) by Sophie Prins, published by Kosmos. Used with permission from the publisher.

Quotes on pp.44, 45, 71 and 163 from *De vader, de moeder & de tijd* (1999) by Marijke Hilhorst, published by Meulenhoff. Used with permission from the author.

Quote on pp.46–7 from *Iris and her friends* (2000) by John Bayley, published by W.W. Norton & Company. Used with permission from W.W. Norton & Company and Gerald Duckworth.

Quote on p.48 from *Dement worden* (1993) by Rien Verdult, published by Hbuitgevers. Used with permission from the publisher.

Quote on pp.51–2 from *Een jaar in scherven* (1987) by Koos van Zomeren, published by Arbeiderspers. Used with permission from the publisher.

Quote on pp.53–4 from *The man with a shattered world* (1992) by A.R. Luria, translated by Lynn Solotoroff, published by Harvard University Press. Used with permission from the publisher.

Quote on p.54 from *Love in the time of cholera* (1988) by Gabriel Marquez, published by Alfred A. Knopf, a division of Random House New York. Used with permission from the publisher.

Quote on pp.59–60 from *De man van de Middenweg* (2001) by Koos van Zomeren, published by Arbeiderspers. Used with permission from the publisher.

Quotes on pp.63 and 69–70 from *Scar Tissue* (1993) by Michael Ignatieff, published by Chattoo & Windus. Used with permission from the Random House Group Ltd.

Quotes on pp.75–6 and 138 from the article *Thuis is ergens anders en nergens meer te vinden* (1990) by Ursula den Tex, published in Vrij Nederland. Used with permission from the author.

Quote on p.100 from *Out of mind* (1988) by J. Bernlef, published by Faber and Faber. Used with permission from the author.

Quote on pp.113–4 from *Elegy for Iris* (1999) by John Bayley, published by St Martin's Press. Used with permission from St Martin's Press and Gerald Duckworth.

Quote on p.122 from in 'Er groeit een nieuwe persoonlijkheid.' In *Het dementiecafé* (2002) edited by Annie van Keymeulen, published by EPO. Used with permission from the publisher.

Quotes on pp.124–5, 144 and 149–50 from *Carien. Het drama van dementie* (1993) by C. Vergoed, published by Uniepers. Used with permission from the daughters of C. Vergoed.

Quotes on pp.133 and 134–5 from *Het verhaal achter de feiten* (1996) by Mia Duijnstee, published by Hbuitgevers. Used with permission from the publisher.

Quote on p.148 from *Meegesleurd in de hel van een Alzheimerpatiënt* (1996) by Willy Wielek, published by Opzij. Used with permission from the publisher.

Quote on pp.150–151 from the article *Alles is goed gekomen.* (1994) by Henk Ruigrok, published in the Nieuwe Revu. Used with permission from the author.

Quote on pp.159–60 from *The story of my father* (2003) by Sue Miller published by Alfred A. Knopf, a division of Random House New York. Used with permission from the publisher.

Contents

Preface

When my father began to show the first signs of impending dementia some 25 years ago, my mother and my brothers and sisters – and I too! – expected that I would be able to clarify for them exactly what was happening to him, and how best we could all deal with it. I had just completed my psycho-gerontology studies (and was therefore an 'expert' on the subject of the psychology of ageing). Despite the fact that I had learned a lot about dementia during the course of my training, it was not at all easy to satisfy the expectations of my mother and my siblings. The illness remained extremely complex, both for my family and for me. This is not only because of the huge number of symptoms such a sickness can manifest – and they can also differ from person to person – but also because the features of the illness change as the sickness progresses. And because the features were devoid of any logic, it was difficult to penetrate its depths, as it were, and to explain why my father's behaviour was different from what it had been in the past.

Slowly but surely, however, I began to discover that there is a simple logic in the signs and symptoms of the disease. It became clear to me that two 'dementia laws', in combination with some basic knowledge of psychology, are sufficient to understand the many deviant behaviour patterns (the dementia symptoms) of this illness. When I explained these two dementia laws to my mother and my brothers and sisters, they were able to understand my father better, and were able to interact with him more effectively.

In the course of many years, I have had the privilege of giving many talks on dementia, for both caregivers in the field and relatives of people with dementia. I have talked about dementia on the basis of the two dementia laws, and after many such lectures I was often asked, by relatives in particular, if my story was available in print. They usually added that they wanted to pass on the information to another relative who had not been able to attend the lecture: 'Then she will also know exactly what is going on, and how to deal with it.' I had to keep on telling them, however, that my story had not yet been published in book form, and I dared not make any promises that it would one day see the light of day in print. And, at first glance, a fairly simple explanation within the context of a talk was one thing, but turning it into a book was something entirely different.

Several papers, by leading experts in the field, have recently appeared in international scientific geriatrics journals that support my simple explanation. This has helped me to step over the threshold of reluctance, and get down at last to producing the book I have been asked to write.

The dementia laws give us a better understanding of what dementia does to its victim, whilst relatives, on the other hand, often want to know what the victim does with the illness; in other words, how does he or she perceive and experience it? I will endeavour to provide an answer to this question in this book.

Dementia creates problems at practically every level of life. It is well-nigh impossible to describe all the problems in great deal and keep the book compact at the same time. I have decided, therefore, to cover 'only' those problems which research has shown present the greatest difficulties for those closest to the person with dementia: communication, mood problems (aggression, depressiveness and suspiciousness), and behaviour problems (clinging behaviour, wandering and nocturnal restlessness).

When one talks with relatives of people with dementia about their worries and their problems, sooner or later the question of guilt will rise to the surface. 'Am I doing it properly?', 'Am I doing enough?', 'If only I had not...' In a book written with family members in particular in mind, the guilt issue cannot be ignored, and this will explain why I have devoted a separate chapter to it.

I have tried to bring the book 'to life' by including a number of quotes, most of which have been taken from (semi)biographical books and interviews. Others (that is, those with no author references) have been drawn from private or work experiences.

1

What is dementia?

Introduction

Her fingers, so wrinkled, the colour of marble, rearrange the advertisement folders lying on the low table.

'What a shame that Pa has just left. It would have been so nice... I don't know where he is, I haven't seen him all day!'

She looks at me with an uncertain expression on her face, grey-blue eyes that look but do not see.

'Pa is making a cup of tea, Mum,' I say as I rest my hand on hers. 'Really? Why didn't he say something then? I haven't seen anything of him at all.'

'Oh, Pa, there you are – that's good.'

She is clearly very pleased to see him. Pa puts the tray with the cups, tea and sugar on the side table. He looks tired.

'Here you are dear, here's the tea,' he says.

She strokes his knee.

'I'm always so pleased when he's back,' she says almost apologetically, and then proceeds to put sugar in all the cups.

(Van den Berg 1995)

The term 'dementia' comes from the Latin and literally means 'mind gone': the first syllable 'de' meaning 'gone', and 'mens' being the Latin word for 'mind'. The person concerned goes into a steady decline, and the progress of the disease is so destructive that in the last phase the patient bears hardly any resemblance to the person he or she was at the outset. During the (long) first phase, the dementia, as such, is scarcely apparent; the eyes are bright and open, the mind is clear and the patient walks and moves around as he has always done. In the final phase of the disorder, however, he becomes dependent on others for all his needs, and he has forgotten everything he has ever learned. A person with severe dementia comes to the end of his life just as he entered it – a helpless baby. At that stage, he is only receptive to the atmosphere around him, and to the satisfaction of his most primary human needs.

It was thought for a long time that people with dementia were 'mad' and suffering from some kind of mental illness. It has become apparent only fairly recently, however, that this is a misconception, and that dementia is caused by brain dysfunction. The nerve cells in the brain are diseased. In the case of Alzheimer's disease, the nerve cells shrink or wither away – in a kind of 'autumn of the mind'. The brain's control room is not able to function as it should. In the early phase of the disease, sufferers are able to behave fairly normally, because most of the nerve cells are still in good working order. The brain also has amazing reserves at its disposal: when nerve cells fail, others take over their tasks, either partly or in whole, and can continue to do so for a very long time...at least until a critical point has been reached, and there are no more 'reserve players waiting on the bench'. The more it affects more parts of the brain, the more striking the changes in the patient's behaviour.

Strictly speaking, a full diagnosis is only possible once a post-mortem examination has been carried out. So long as the patient is still alive, there is no reliable method of determining the nature and degree of the brain tissue damage. Dementia, therefore, is always a 'probable' diagnosis. And sometimes, even the most experienced pathologists are puzzled by the fact that some people who have apparently functioned quite normally for their entire lives are found, during autopsy, to have the same brain abnormality as that found in people with dementia. This means that, even after death, it is not possible in all cases to diagnose Alzheimer's disease with 100 per cent certainty.

The disease begins gradually: silent, like an animal stalking its night-time prey, it takes hold of its victim, and worsens with time.

Dementia in many forms

There are many types of dementia, and dementia – like cancer, rheumatism and respiratory disorders – is a collective term. The most common form of the illness is Alzheimer's disease, which is named after the German neurologist Alois Alzheimer, who first described it in 1906.

The first conversation Alois Alzheimer had with Auguste D., the 'first' Alzheimer patient, began as follows:

'What is your name?'
'Auguste.'
'Your surname?'
'Auguste.'
'What is your husband's name?'
'Auguste, I think.'
'Your husband?'
'Ah, my husband.'

She looks at me as if she has not quite understood the
question.
    'Are you married?'
    'To Auguste.'
    'Mrs D.?'
    'Yes, Auguste D.'
    'How long have you been married?'
    She is obviously trying hard to remember.
    'Three weeks.'

Of all people suffering from dementia, roughly 55 per cent
have Alzheimer's in its purest form. After Alzheimer's, vascular
dementia is the most common and is responsible for 15 per
cent of all dementia cases. There are other forms of vascular
dementia, the most well-known being the so-called multi-
infarct dementia (MID). As the name suggests, this dementia
arises from the many (in Latin: multi) small brain infarcts that
cause oxygen loss in various parts of the brain which, in its turn,
results in brain tissue erosion.

In roughly 15 per cent of cases, we see a combination of
two or more disorders which lead ultimately to dementia. The
combination of Alzheimer's and vascular dementia occurs most
frequently. If we add 'pure Alzheimer dementia' to the 15 per
cent mentioned above, it means that roughly 70 per cent of all
dementia patients suffer from Alzheimer's disease.

A long line of relatively rare disorders is responsible for the
remaining 15 per cent. These diseases, including Parkinson's
disease Pick's disease, Binswanger disease, Lewy Body disease
and Huntington's disease, occur – relatively speaking – more
often in younger patients. The same is true of Aids which, in its
last phase, can also cause dementia.

Dementia is a syndrome; that is, a group of symptoms or
features which appear in combination. Memory loss is always

the essence of the illness, and it means in practice that the patient's life pattern undergoes considerable change. As we have said already, there are many types of dementia. Each syndrome has its own cause, or causes, and each has its own process. We will limit ourselves in this chapter to a description of the two most common forms of dementia: Alzheimer's disease and MID.

Both diseases share many similarities, in terms of their symptoms and consequences. There are, however, several important differences. Whilst Alzheimer develops very slowly, MID often begins suddenly with a period of confusion, which is probably the consequence of a mild stroke. This is followed by a period of reasonable recovery, the patient's condition remaining fairly stable until the onset of the next 'confusion' period. Whilst Alzheimer progresses in a way which can be compared to walking down a slight slope, MID is more reminiscent of small steps on a descending track – two steps down, and one upward step back, and so on.

Because MID is caused by the erosion of many small brain particles, whereby the surrounding area is still able to function reasonably well, these patients are often far longer aware of their own deterioration than Alzheimer patients. When someone with Alzheimer's disease makes a mistake of some kind, and this is pointed out to him, his response is often one of genuine surprise. The recent past is a black hole for him, whilst a similar incident might ring a few more bells for an MID patient, who realizes quite quickly, or remembers vaguely, what he should have known. MID patients are likely to be more conscious of the effects of their illness for a longer period of time.

A male MID patient describes his experiences in these terms:

I used to be able to do everything. And now I can't do anything. That's what's so crazy about all this. Everything works against me. If I had my way…I would walk through that wall, get into the car, and go to see my wife. But I can't. If I could, I would have done it already! And that's what gets me down. I can't stand it. I cannot cope without my wife. And here I am [in the nursing home]. That's all I know. I don't understand it. Everything is confused. I don't know what's going on any more. And I can't remember how it was in the past. There is so much I would like to know…and I know nothing, that's the whole problem. The fact of the matter is: I can't remember anything. There is nothing I can do about it, but what I know this morning, I will know this afternoon…I don't know any more. That is horrible. They say to me: 'go and get ten kilos of potatoes' – and a moment later, I'm saying to myself: what was it I was supposed to get? And then I've lost it. I used to know exactly what I had to do, but now I don't.

My brother-in-law was here a while ago. I think to myself: 'hey, that's Gerard'. I was happy to see him, of course, because we grew up and played together. He says: 'You ought to be able to remember that, Henk.' I say: 'Yes, I ought to, but I can't, Gerard.'

I'm not doing anyone any harm, and no one is harming me, but I lose track of things immediately. How can I get rid of this illness? – because in my eyes it is an illness.

But enough of this self-pity. That's no good. I will keep on fighting. I'll just eat a plum, and then at least I'll have something to nibble on in my mouth.

(Quoted in Van Delft 1993)

The fact that people with dementia are spectators of their own decline over a longer period of time often results in their developing depression.

Whenever the term 'dementia' is used, it usually refers not so much to MID but to Alzheimer's disease. Unless otherwise stated, therefore, the same will be true of the rest of this book.

Prevalence

Dementia is often referred to as the 'disease of old age', although the disorder is occasionally known to occur in people under the age of 65 years. Between the ages of 45 and 54, however, only 0.025 per cent of the population suffers from dementia. The incidence figure is still less than 1 per cent in the 65-year-old age group, although between the ages of 65 and 70 it rises to 2.5 per cent. After that, the percentage doubles every five years. The illness is thus particularly prevalent among the very old; 1 in 5 of those aged 85 and over suffers from dementia. In order to emphasize that dementia is not always the inevitable consequence of reaching a grand old age, it is worth formulating the last sentence in more positive terms: that is, four out of every five octogenarians *escape dementia.*

Increased life-expectancy has resulted in a sharp rise in the number of dementia patients in recent years, and the upward trend is unlikely to end in the foreseeable future. Dementia has already become one of the top five causes of death in the Western world, and in consequence is sometimes referred to as the 'disease of the century'.

Causes

All kinds of reasons have been put forward through the years which might explain why dementia occurs. One popular explanation which reigned for a long time was that the brain had been damaged by a virus. Another explanation is metal poisoning, aluminium in particular (in drinking water). A third explanation seeks it in the neurotransmitter acetylcholine, a chemical substance essential to the working of the brain.

The profusion of explanations makes one thing very clear indeed, however: the precise cause of dementia is not known. Despite this, there is no doubt at all that genetic factors play a role in the development of the disease. Research has already proven that the (immediate) relatives of people with dementia are twice as likely as others to develop dementia. The same is also true for relatives of people with Down's syndrome – they too have an increased chance of developing dementia. The fact that dementia primarily occurs in older people suggests that ageing also plays a role.

Finally, it is also known that there is a higher risk of dementia occurring in people who have suffered a severe skull trauma at some time in their lives, and in those with chronic high blood pressure. As far as the latter is concerned, increased blood pressure not only raises the chances of vascular dementia, but doubles the chances of developing Alzheimer's disease as well.

There is no need for immediate panic if we appear to fall into one or more of the above-mentioned risk categories; the chances of our *not* developing dementia are still much higher than the chances of our being struck down by it.

2

The simple logic behind dementia

Introduction

Living with, and caring for, a partner/relative with dementia is often far from easy. The patient's behaviour is often very puzzling for those around him: he constantly asks the same questions; he can remember nothing about recent events, but is very lucid about the distant past; he wants to go home when he is already there; he plays with dolls but feels very insulted if he is spoken to as a child; he forgets everything but never admits to being forgetful; and so on. What confuses people around him most is the unpredictability of his current behaviour.

There is a simple logic in the symptoms of his illness, nonetheless. Two 'dementia laws', in combination with some degree of simple psychological knowledge, are sufficient for us to be able to understand the many anomalous aspects of his behaviour – that is, the dementia symptoms. We will try to throw some light on this aspect in this chapter.

How we remember

To be able to explain the first of these dementia laws, we need first of all to say something about how the normal memory mechanism works (see Figure 2.1). Scientists have discovered that, generally speaking, we humans have two kinds of memory: a short-term and a long-term memory. Everything we hear, see, taste, smell or feel (the five senses), at any given moment, enters our short-term memory first. This information stays in this small anteroom of our upper chamber for no more than 20 or 30 seconds. Within the space of half a minute, therefore, we have to make a selection. Important information receives our attention and the rest we discard. If we want to increase the retention period, the information will have to be transferred to our long-term memory chamber, the large warehouse which, in everyday language, we call 'the memory'.

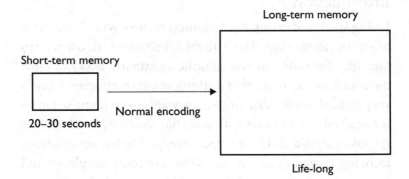

Figure 2.1 Normal encoding

Whilst the short-term memory has a very small capacity, our long-term memory gives us enough space in which to 'store' endless quantities of information. It is never 'full'. By comparison, the largest of our modern-day computers can offer no more information storage space than would fill just one piece of paper. A second and pleasing feature of this large memory of ours is that it is 'life-long'; that is, it retains all the information it receives throughout the entire course of our lives.

Transporting, or the *encoding* of, information from the short-term to the long-term memory is not an automatic process. It requires effort. Studies have shown that various factors play a role in our process of memorizing. One extremely important factor is attention. What, we may ask, has the greatest influence on the ability to concentrate our attention? Emotions, both pleasing and unpleasing. A highly emotional event stays with us all our lives. Not all information touches us emotionally. Dull and 'dry' information, however, can also be retained for a longer period of time, provided we exercise extra effort in 'holding' it. A classic way of memorizing is repetition. It is not so long ago that children learned new words at school by repeating them out loud, again and again.

Our memory is not only helped by repetition, but also by our ability to visualize. Information which we absorb from a picture held in front of us (*visualization*) is more readily retained. If the Chinese proverb is true, then 'a picture says more than a thousand words'.

We can also remember things better if we can *associate* them with something else. Memory wizards often hang new information on the hatstand of old information. Even the less intellectual among us, however, are able to retain information by relating it to something we already know.

The more you know about a certain subject, the more successful you will be in absorbing even more about it. If you know a great deal about computers, for instance, you will remember much more of what you have read in a newspaper article, or have seen on television, about the latest developments in the computer field, than you would if you were hitherto totally ignorant of the subject.

Another way of retaining something in the memory is to keep our information structures in proper order. If you were asked to remember the words 'pear', 'gull', 'peach', 'goose' and 'gannet', you would probably have some difficulty in doing so, especially if you regard them as purely separate words, independent of each other. The task becomes much easier, however, if you divide the five words into two categories: two kinds of fruit (both beginning with a 'p') and three bird species (each beginning with a 'g').

Your capacity to remember something is largely dependent on whether the information has *meaning* for you. You will remember far less of a conversation between two foreigners in a foreign language than you would of a conversation between two compatriots in your own language.

A good teacher will endeavour to add a touch of *humour* to his lessons. Information given with a very straight face will be much less likely to 'stick in the mind' than it would if it were served up in a humourous 'sauce'.

To summarize – the memory process is particularly helped by the following factors:

- attention
- repetition
- making something visual or visualization
- association
- keeping the memory 'files' in proper order
- meaningful information
- humour.

This overview of the memory has made it clear that remembering information is not a process that runs automatically. You have to work at it, even though you may not always be aware of your own input during the actual process of encoding.

The first law of dementia: disturbed encoding

We have now reached the stage of being able to unveil the first law of dementia (see Figure 2.2). If someone has dementia (that is, as a result of Alzheimer's disease), he is no longer able to transport information from his short-term memory to his long-term memory. His ability to absorb information is disturbed, and it means in practice that he can no longer remember what was happening around him a mere 30 seconds ago.

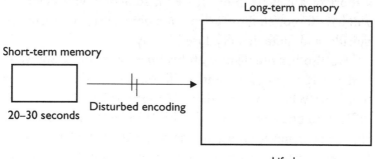

Figure 2.2 Disturbed encoding

However, people never behave 100 per cent according to the norm, and here, too, there is an exception to the rule. If information evokes many emotions, or is repeated frequently, it might be possible for the person with dementia to absorb at least some of it. He might, for instance, be able to remember hearing his GP say something about a nursing home during a recent visit – and he remembers it because it touched, and still touches, a very tender nerve in him. A well-known fact is that people with dementia who are collected by bus every morning and taken to a day centre will know in the course of time that the bus will arrive at their front door in the morning.

Direct consequences

The phenomenon of disturbed encoding enables us to understand many features of dementia. The signs of early dementia, in particular, are now quite easy to explain.

One of the first symptoms of the disorder is that the person can no longer travel in an area new and unknown to him. Just like any other person, someone with a mild form of dementia walking through the streets of an unfamiliar town will try to memorize a number of orientation points such as a street name, a shop, or a church spire. However, someone with dementia will have forgotten those orientation points very soon. He will quickly, and quite literally, lose his way.

He also has problems with his time-orientation. Someone in the early stages of dementia will constantly ask: 'What's the time?', or 'What day is it today – Monday or Tuesday?' It is not difficult to guess the reason for this. Time does not stand still; change is its most important characteristic. In order to know the time, you have to look at your watch, or clock, several times a day – and then 'print' the hours and minutes in your head. When this fails, however, the time of day represents a constant puzzle.

Early-stage dementia patients can bring those around them close to despair by asking the same question over and over again. When a short period of time has passed, they cannot remember having asked the question in the first place, let alone their having been given an answer to it. For the same reason, they play the same CD several times a day, and tell the same story while doing so.

The English author Linda Grant writes about her mother who has dementia:

> Apart from the physical wasting, the diminution of her body to the size of a large doll, she looked normal – she

looked like a sweet little old lady – and people would start up conversations with her which would proceed as they expected until a question answered a moment before would be asked again – 'No, I must interrupt, you haven't told me yet where you live.'

'As I just said, Birmingham.' And then asked and asked until you lost your patience because you thought you had been entering a dialogue which had its rules of exchange, and it turned our that what you were really talking to was an animate brick wall. Questions asked over and over again not because she couldn't remember the reply but because a very short tape playing in her head had reached its end and wound itself back to the beginning to start afresh. She knew the conventions of conversations – these had not deserted her – but she could not recall what she had said herself a few moments before.

Sometimes the question was repeated before the person she was asking had finished getting through their response.

There were little holes in her brain, real holes in the grey matter, where the memory of her life used to be, and of what she had done half an hour or even a few minutes ago.

(Grant 1998)

Many relatives give another reason for no longer being able to have a reasonable conversation with their father or uncle who have dementia: 'He doesn't listen to anything I say. I'm in the middle of my story, and he suddenly interrupts and starts talking about something entirely different. That's very exhausting.' The person in question, however, cannot help it. If a story lasts for more than 30 seconds, he soon loses track of it because he has already forgotten the first all-important sentences which opened the 'conversation'. He steps, as it were, into a film which began some time ago. It is not surprising, then, that his attention wanes somewhat after he has done his best to listen to someone for a few moments, and that he suddenly switches to another subject. And this is also why people with dementia lose their interest in reading newspapers or books.

Family members have even more reasons to complain when they find that their relative with dementia is no longer able to join in a conversation about an event from the recent past. He cannot even provide answers to simple questions such as: 'What did you have for breakfast today?', or 'Did the children visit you yesterday?' His disturbed encoding capacity also means that he is scarcely able to absorb any new information at all.

The partner of a man with mild dementia illustrates this point:

> When the front door of our house ceased to function properly after a break-in, we had no choice but to install a new lock. However, the mechanism of the new lock was different from the old one. My husband, who customarily locked the door each evening before going to bed, was now very bad tempered every evening because he didn't know how it worked any more.

As soon as the Big Forget begins, so too (usually) does the Big Search. The person with dementia is constantly losing things, because he cannot remember where he left them. Furthermore, because in this 'foggy' stage of the dementia he puts even greater value on his possessions than he did in the past, he will try even harder to put them away in a safe place. The result is that he then spends a large part of his time looking for them. Someone once said in jest: the only positive thing to be said about dementia is that the patient can now hide his own slipper before playing 'Hunt the Slipper'!

Because of the faulty encoding process, people with dementia all too quickly develop problems in recognizing or remembering people new to them; that is, those who have only recently entered their lives. This can be a very painful experience. Such as for the young girl whose boyfriend has accompanied her five times already on her visits to her grandfather, who, even on the sixth visit, still asks: 'Tell me, who is that young man you have brought with you today?'

We use our long-term memory not only to 'hold' the details of past events in our heads; we also need it on a day-to-day basis in order to know what we must do now, later, next week, or next month. In other words, our memory also serves as a kind of diary in that it contains our future plans, important dates and appointments, and the birthdays of friends and family.

A partner/relative with dementia forgets his intentions and plans, because they no longer reach the mainland of his long-term memory. (A second reason for people with dementia not being able to remember appointments lies in the disorientation in time which we mentioned earlier; that is, they no longer know what day it is today.) Dementia, therefore, not only causes the recent past to disintegrate, but the future too.

If a person who does not suffer from dementia is angry with someone and has a good reason for that anger – he has, perhaps, just been unjustly accused of something – it is unlikely that he will saunter down the road whistling a happy tune five minutes later. His unhappy mood will hover in the air for some time to come. One of the reasons for this is that he wants to show others that he really meant what he said. People suffering from dementia however, are subject to much more fluctuating moods, and they very quickly forget what lay behind their anger, sorrow, shame or joy. When they are laughing, they will have forgotten that five minutes earlier they were feeling very unhappy indeed. And then we tend to say: 'They are just like small children.'

The reader will now understand why some dementia sufferers will go to the same local shop several times a day, and bring back the same items in his shopping bag.

Here then are the direct consequences of the disturbed encoding:

- disorientation in an unfamiliar environment
- disorientation in time
- the same questions are asked repeatedly
- the same story is told repeatedly
- the patient quickly loses track of things
- the patient is unable to answer any questions about recent events
- the patient is unable to learn anything new
- the patient quickly loses things
- disorientation in respect of people new to him
- appointments are quickly forgotten
- mood swings are frequent.

Indirect consequences

In the early stages of dementia especially, people with dementia are often perfectly aware that they are making mistakes and that they are able to do less than they used to. They notice too that they are less able to cope with the new and the unfamiliar. They 'bump their heads', as it were, on this wall of reduced capacity, they botch things and they grind to a complete halt because of the gaps in their memory – and all this, several times a day.

New faces, an unfamiliar setting, friends who ask about something that happened recently – someone with dementia knows that situations like these will bring uneasy and embarrassing moments with them. We do not need a vast amount of psychological knowledge to realize, therefore, that because of this people with dementia will do everything in their power to avoid such occasions. One of the early signs is that the person will prefer to stay at home and avoid occasions which will bring them into contact with people they do not know well. Protecting their own private space limits the number of mistakes and blunders. In order not to make mistakes, they undertake far less, and show less initiative, than they might have done a decade or two earlier. To this we have to add the fact that they also quickly forget what they had in mind. For some dementia sufferers, doing nothing at all is their enduring occupation.

People who do not suffer from dementia will often try to hide or camouflage faults they make in the company of others. Like all of us, the dementia patient also knows that to err is human. Confronted by their own errors, they might find themselves lying to someone – something they probably would never have done before. In order to sustain their precious self-esteem, some people with dementia can even become extremely adept at thinking up all kinds of 'white' lies and excuses. A Chinese proverb suggests that if we humans could see ourselves, in terms of our human traits, as an onion which we peel away, layer by layer, all that would remain would be our pride. A person with dementia will want to keep the façade of his 'house' looking good, in order to lure others into believing that the inside of the house is in equally excellent order. Instead of all those 'white' lies, someone with dementia may also retreat into conjuring up 'avoidance', and often very shrewd, answers. If you ask him what he had for breakfast this morning, he might say 'Oh, the same as always', or 'Since when have you been interested in what I had for breakfast?' We find a very good example of a 'shrewd' answer in the children's novel *Memory* by the New Zealand writer Margaret Mahy (1987):

> She filled two cups with water, untainted by tea. Johnny accepted his with relief rather than disappointment, but Sophie sat peering into her own cup, aware that something was not quite right.
>
> 'It's very weak,' she said dubiously.

Because the encoding process is disturbed, and because the reality confronting someone with dementia is so painful, he often comes to believe his own fantasies. Many people with dementia forget that they are forgetful. They believe their memories are working well, and they will adamantly deny any disorder.

Another strategy often used when such patients are married or live with their children is that by secretly thinking up all kinds of excuses or reasons along the way, they shift more and more tasks onto the family members in the house, the partner or the daughter(-in-law) especially, who then respond by complaining about the patient's laziness, apathy, indifference and lack of initiative – at least, as long as they are still unaware of the true nature of his condition. Whatever it may be, the most important person in the patient's immediate environment becomes the essential guide who will take him through the 'landscape' of his life, which is becoming increasingly strange to him; and in order not to lose his way, he follows her around like a child.

It seems, from the fact that the partner/relative with dementia knows who the key person is for him and, therefore, does not want to let him or her out of his sight, that he knows deep inside himself that there is something fundamentally wrong with him. Something is churning inside him, and anxiety or impending anxiety is never far away. How do we respond to anxiety? How do we respond to an enormous calamity which is taking place inside us? The answer is that this depends on the person's individual character or personality. One will become aggressive, the other depressive, and the third suspicious, and so on. Some who, before the onset of the illness, tended in times of setback to put the blame for the mishap on others will do the same now, and will be more inclined to show anger towards others for errors committed. This kind of person can become a real 'grouch' for those around him.

Another response in the onset phase of dementia is the emergence of suspicious behaviour. 'I am not at fault, but others are making life difficult for me by doing nasty things behind my back.' The subject of his suspicion is nearly always someone in his immediate environment: his partner, the daughter who is caring for him, the Help the Aged home-help, the social nurse, the ward orderly.

A frequently occurring reaction to the early stages of dementia is depressiveness, which occurs particularly in those who have always had a tendency towards self-doubt. In the face of setbacks they will now feel – as they have always done – that they have no one but themselves to blame. 'I'm hopeless. I can't do anything right.'

Other possible reactions to frustration or existential anxiety include: the hoarding of food or goods (inwardly they feel the impending threat of their own disintegration, and they therefore prepare themselves for the bad times that lie ahead); physical restlessness and nervous behaviour, for example pacing back and forth, or unable any longer to sit quietly in a chair; and excessive eating, drinking or smoking or, conversely, a total refusal to accept any further intakes of food or fluids. It has to be said, however, that these psychological reactions are not characteristic solely of people with dementia. They manifest themselves in normal people too, particularly those battling with the emotional pain or anxiety following the loss of someone dear to them. In this sense, the psychological functioning of someone with dementia is not so much 'odd' as very normal.

Many people with dementia do not limit themselves to just one of the response possibilities given above, but to several. Some, for instance, swing from anger to depression, others combine hoarding behaviour with restlessness, whilst others can be extremely passive and dependent: in this case, the only activity is eating and smoking.

Someone in the early stages of dementia not only responds normally to anxiety and uncertainty – his other behaviour traits will also be no different from ours. We too are capable of getting lost in a place we do not know, losing a key, forgetting an appointment, responding aggressively or depressively to fear or a severe setback, becoming suspicious when something goes wrong and we have forgotten that we played a role in it, and so on. The difference between us and our partner/relative with dementia is that we only occasionally make mistakes or react differently to them, whilst for someone with dementia they happen continuously.

The indirect consequences of disturbed encoding can be summarized as follows:

- contact avoidance, withdrawal
- loss of initiative
- façade erection: lies and (shrewd) evasion of questions

- denial of being forgetful
- dependency, even 'claiming' at times
- aggression, depressiveness, suspiciousness
- hoarding
- physical restlessness (pacing back and forth)
- excessive eating, drinking or smoking.

The second law of dementia: the roll-back memory

> 'Here I am again,' she said to her mother. 'How are you feeling now?'
>
> Her mother looked up. 'Thank you,' she said politely, in a high-pitched, slightly shrill, voice – 'but I want to go to my children now.'
>
> 'But you are with your children, Mum.'
>
> Her mother looked surprised: 'Am I with my children?'
>
> 'Yes, we are your children, aren't we?'
>
> (Voskuil 1999)

The features of the early stages of dementia can be reasonably well explained on the basis of the first law of dementia, although it will not suffice to explain what we are able to observe in mild and severe dementia; for this, we need the second law. In order to explain what it contains, however, we first of all have to say, once again, something about the normal, healthy, memory.

We can imagine the long-term memory as a large library stacked full with personal diaries, or in the words of the Irish writer Oscar Wilde: 'Memory...is the diary that we all carry about with us.' Anyone with an efficiently-working brain might want to write everything he feels is worthwhile in his 'mental' diary. The Dutch journalist and writer Willem Oltmans, for instance, managed to fill 250,000 diary pages over a period of 40 years; that is almost 18 pages a day.

Each one of us, in fact, works – unnoticed – on a 'mental' diary of events and thoughts that put Oltmans' work completely in the shade; we fill these diaries with all kinds of items which, for one reason or another, we feel deserve to be written down.

Here is a small, random, miscellany: a tonsil operation; the arrival of a baby sister; the manners our parents taught us; games with Grandpa; Granny's death; the first day at school; learning to read and write at primary school; geography knowledge; inhaled scents and smells; falling in love; meaningful discussions and encounters; the countless big and small successes and disappointments; becoming a parent. We fill thousands of these memory diaries in the course of our lives. If we are going to be able to call on our memory to deliver quickly the particular diary we need at any given moment, it is essential that the whole collection is properly stacked on the shelves, and in proper sequence, year by year.

Someone in his eighties who has been suffering from dementia for the last three years will remember very little of what has happened in that period of time. His disturbed memory processes have made it impossible for him to 'write' any diaries in those three years. The last three volumes on the shelf, therefore, are empty. He will be well able, nonetheless, to tell all sorts of stories about the people and events of his (long) pre-dementia life – that is, before he reached the age of 77 years.

This changes as the dementia relentlessly advances – and this is when we see the second law of dementia in action. The long-term memory begins to disintegrate, and in a very striking way: it rolls up, as it were, beginning with the most recent and ending with the most distant, step by step (see Figure 2.3). The first diaries to disappear are those that were 'written' a year before the onset of the dementia, followed by the year before that, and so on. We cannot escape the comparison with the book-worm penetrating into our memory library and nibbling at our diaries. These animals have a preference for fresh food, and this will explain why they start chomping their way into the most recent of the diaries. The last to go are the childhood memories. In the very advanced stage

The memory of a 77-year-old without dementia – the shelf on which the diaries containing the memories of his entire life are stacked is still intact.

Years

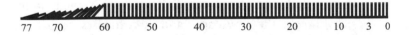

| 77 | 70 | 60 | 50 | 40 | 30 | 20 | 10 | 3 | 0 |

The memory of a 77-year-old patient with dementia who has lost his memories of the last 17 years – the diaries begin to collapse, first the most recent, then those preceding them, and so on.

Years

| 77 | 70 | 60 | 50 | 40 | 30 | 20 | 10 | 3 | 0 |

The memory of someone in the advanced stage of dementia – only the memories of his early childhood remain.

Years

| 77 | 70 | 60 | 50 | 40 | 30 | 20 | 10 | 3 | 0 |

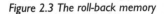

Figure 2.3 The roll-back memory

of dementia, therefore, the patient is left with nothing more than the diaries of the first five years of his life; in the final phase, even these disappear, and very soon after that the patient dies.

There are two exceptions to the second – that is, the disappearing diaries – dementia law. The first, and the less pleasing of the two, is that the diaries containing more complex information are swallowed up in the thick and all-consuming mists of dementia, sooner than one might expect, in fact, on the basis of the roll-back memory concept. They are the kind of diaries that might include such subjects as: calculations and bookkeeping; cooking; solving difficult problems; organizing a party; repairing a bike, etc. What is complex is also something that differs from person to person, and it depends entirely on the individual's own talents and interests.

Here we have the story of the partner of someone with dementia (a one-time economics lawyer) who sees guests at his table who are not there:

> To move with him into his shadowy world is the simplest thing to do, and it creates the least tension. Fortunately, it is not necessary to enter into conversation with the other guests, and once 'the guests' have been served, John simply reads the newspaper and does his best to gather wisdom from what is going on in the world. Surprisingly enough, the economy section and the Stock Exchange fluctuations continue, as always, to grab his interest. He is also able to offer some very sensible comments on top managerial sackings and shifts taking place in national corporations in response to current problems.
>
> With increasing amazement, I listen to his personal viewpoints, his well-founded and well-formulated judgement of certain matters, but am unable to reconcile

them with his strange 'host-behaviour'. Why does something like this happen? Where are things going wrong in his brain? Why is he able to make intelligent statements on executive board policies, and at the same time is alarmed by the presence of invisible guests around him? What he is saying now sounds perfectly reasonable, doesn't it? Just as it was and just as it has always been?

(Prins 1997)

The second exception is a more pleasing one. Diaries which contain vast quantities of words (repetition) remain accessible for a longer period of time. It is as if the book-worms we met a short while ago are reluctant to begin their feast, because they fear they might be interrupted too often. Diary records of significant events, good or bad, are also spared the destruction process for longer. An example of this is the death by drowning of the favourite grandchild ten years before.

The consequences

The comparison with the disappearing diaries gives a useful insight into the many behaviour patterns of someone in the last stages of dementia. The blurring of the memory means that at a certain moment he will no longer be able to exercise the (instrumental) skills he spent the last 15 or 20 years of his life learning. A dementia patient passing beyond the mild dementia stage will inevitably, in the course of time, have problems with the coffee-maker. The day will come when the diary containing instructions on how to use today's modern kitchen equipment has disappeared and, in the face of it, our patient will decide to put the coffee-maker aside, fill a saucepan with water, place it on the gas, and then spoon some coffee into it. This means that because he no longer has access to all the know-how and skills he has learned in, say, the last two decades, he now has no choice but to fall back on earlier habits.

It is also possible, therefore, that one day he will start sweeping the carpet with a dustpan and brush because he no longer knows how to use the vacuum cleaner. Another possibility is that instead of using the washing machine he will start filling the sink with water and soap, and do the washing just as his grandmother did before him; assuming, of course, that he still has the energy, and the opportunity, to do it.

The crumbling memory also has the effect of putting important biographical information out of the patient's reach. He will forget, for instance, that he is retired, and will want to go to work. Relatives responsible for the care of such patients will sometimes have to develop a whole spectrum of strategies, tricks and persuasion techniques, in order to prevent the patient from embarrassing himself and his family; for example, by suddenly turning up again in the office now occupied by his successor of many years.

The day will also dawn when he will no longer see his own house as his.

> Mr Jones is very forgetful. For the last 15 years, he and his wife have lived together in a sheltered accommodation in the centre of the town. I help them with their housework three times a week, and if the weather permits I always take Mr Jones for a short walk. One day something strange happens. When we reach his house after our walk, he stops and asks: 'Where are you taking me to? You are surely not going to ring the bell here – I don't know this house.' It catches me unawares and I am not sure what to do. And then I remember what had been said during a dementia course I followed some time ago: when the illness worsens, the patient may not recognize his own home and will want to go back to the house he lived in

some years back. I suddenly have a brainwave. I bend over and whisper into his ear: 'Mr Jones, let's just ring the bell because I believe your wife is here.' He agrees to this, and when he sees his wife opening the door he flies into her arms, and with emotion in his voice he says: 'What are you doing here?'

(A home-help)

Dementia also goes hand in hand with a disappearing awareness of how we should behave in the company of others.

I always used to enjoy going for a meal with my husband, but I dare not do it any more. He makes improper comments to the waiter, and I feel terribly uncomfortable when I see the people at the other tables give us disapproving looks as my husband noisily shovels his food, *sans* knife and fork, into his mouth. He feels no embarrassment at entering into discussion, and arguing, with total strangers. He would never have done that before.

(A wife)

People do not, by nature, act according to the behaviour norms of the day; they only do so after a long and difficult process of learning what society has decided is good and not good. As the 'social behaviour' diaries fade into the mist, loss of decorum follows. No matter in what company he finds himself, the person with dementia will in no way be deterred from picking his nose, burping, breaking wind, slopping food down himself, noisily slurping his drink, walking around with open 'flies', urinating wherever it pleases him, waving to total strangers, and so forth.

We are not born with words in our mouth. The ability to articulate, and to compile a comprehensive vocabulary, plus a reasonable knowledge of grammar, entails – in the same way as behaviour norms – a learning process spread over many years. The older we get, the better we learn to speak our mother-tongue, and if all is well we can even improve on it well into our seventies. Our language memory, therefore, is not confined to one diary, but to many hundreds, all contained in the 'Annual Editions' stored in our library. Our ability, via language, to communicate does not suddenly disappear, therefore; it happens very gradually. The first signs are problems finding words, so that 'What do you call that thing?' becomes an ever-recurring question put by patients with dementia to those around them.

An old lady in the early stages of dementia says:

> When we come back from Church, we will wait until everyone is back, and then we'll all sit down together. I like that! Mother will have the coffee ready, and she always pours a good cup of coffee. Mother is a good cook and makes very good coffee. And then it's just like being in a hotel…HAHAHA…that's nice, isn't it? She always keeps a separate – what's it called? – saucepan! Or something like that. Wonderful. She prepares it all herself. She can make wonderful soups too and also – what do you call those things you throw up into the air… In the air? They can often fall to the ground and break, and I've done that a few times.
>
> (Quoted in Van Delft 1993)

This search for the right words often means that conversations become slower and more difficult than normal; *too* slow and *too* difficult for many dementia patients. It is no surprise, then, that they make less and less effort to talk about anything at all. In the final phase of dementia, even the most devoted of relatives and carers will be unable to enter into any degree of conversation with the patient, for the simple reason that his language library, which was once so comprehensive, has shrivelled to no more than a few words. The ability to converse has now reached the level of a toddler. Many patients in this phase of dementia – like the toddler they once were learning to speak – repeat words or sentences they hear others saying. Some dementia patients are ultimately unable to speak at all. But before that stage is reached, it is quite possible for the person concerned to switch over to the language he spoke as a child. Someone who has spoken standard English for most of his life might, as a result of his crumbling memory, for instance, return to the dialect he grew up with in order to express himself.

The situation is even more difficult for a Turkish immigrant, for instance, ending his days in a Dutch nursing home, or a Polish immigrant in a geriatric home in England. Those patients not living in the land of their birth become isolated because there is no one around them who understands their language.

Another drama in the dementing process is that at a certain moment we see that the patient is unable to recognize his or her own spouse. The diaries containing the date of his wedding, and memories of his 'courting' days before it, have all gone.

> A month ago I was washing him and he said: 'I'll just call Carla.' And I'm Carla. It gave me quite a shock. He didn't recognize me any more – his own wife. The children and our GP had warned me that this could happen, but it still knocked me for six. And it has happened several times since then. This morning, he said: 'You look just like Carla – that's nice!'
>
> (A wife)

The moment will come too when the patient's own children will be strangers for him.

> She asked her younger son, Marcel, who has grown into a heavily-built man, now almost 30 years of age, whether he and Sjaak were brothers. She points to the older of the two, who is a little shorter and darker-skinned than Marcel. 'Yes,' Marcel replies, 'we are brothers, and we are your sons. We are your children.' She is prepared to accept the fact that they are brothers, but that they are her sons, let alone her children, is going too far.
>
> She laughs heartily: 'Oh, no, you can't fool me. Big men like you can't be children.'
>
> At the cemetery, Mother admires the lovely trees, 'so thick too', and the colourful plants on the graves, 'it looks like a flower shop', she says…until it slowly dawns on her where she is. She asks softly what a cemetery actually is, and whose grave Pa is working on. She then asks her elder daughter: 'Are your mother and father buried here?'
>
> (Hilhorst 1999)

The loss of the partner will often be 'compensated' for by bringing 'back to life' various people who have been dead for many years.

> The telephone rings and my wife answers it with the words: 'Hello, this is Orpington 99406, can I help you?' It is, in fact, the telephone number of the house she had worked in as a maid 60 years before.
>
> (A husband)

People who played an important role in an earlier part of the patient's life are more likely to be 'resurrected', and for most it will be the parents.

Mother and Father have recently been given a place at the lunch table in the home together with the noisy eaters, the dribblers, the toothless, the slurpers and the spitters. The staff call this table 'The Ritz Hotel'. Sometimes, I join the lunch guests at table, as I did on this day in autumn.

Father slips the meat he has just cut into small pieces into his jacket pocket: 'It's tough, so where else can I put it?' Mother is given finely minced food because she is not able to chew very well. Father feels he has to sit at this table for Mother's sake, but he is not at all happy about it. They bicker a bit, and suddenly Mother says: 'If you go on like this, I'll just say: Hilhorst, I've had enough of this, and I'm leaving.'

'Where will you go?' I ask.

'Oh, to my mother, of course.'

(Hilhorst 1999)

There is no logic to disappearing diaries. When an older person with dementia looks into the mirror, he might not recognize his own reflection. Perhaps he is thinking: 'I don't know that old man with the wrinkled face and grey hair.' He believes he is much younger than the face looking out at him from the mirror. It might be that he sees the image as his long-dead father; he might even see his daughter as his wife.

Memory serves as a kind of glue for the personality, the characteristics which typify us as individuals. When our memory falls away, the core of the person we once were also crumbles. Our own behaviour patterns, together with the set lines which link our thoughts, our feelings and our behaviour – and which we have made our own over the course of the years – are broken.

Outsiders often notice, therefore, that the person with dementia is behaving 'strangely'; that is, differently and unexpectedly. You might often hear a dementia patient's partner or child say something like: 'I don't recognize them any more. They have changed so much.'

Another very conspicuous aspect of dementia is the patient's deteriorating ability to look after himself properly. People with dementia will tend to carry out all the necessary self-care activities in the opposite sequence to the way they learned them. The dementia patient with a pure form of Alzheimer's disease (and no added illnesses) will start to have difficulties in carrying out complicated tasks such as cooking, shopping and finances. In a later phase he will be unable to choose a proper selection of clothing for the day (for example, two vests, one brown sock, one blue sock, etc.), and it may often take considerable persuasion to get him to take a shower.

In a subsequent phase, he will not be able to dress himself without help, and later he will need help to bath and wash himself, and later again he will no longer remember what is required to go to the toilet. He will then become incontinent for urine and, later, for faeces.

The erosion process of memory doesn't stop at this point, because there inevitably comes a time when the patient needs assistance with eating and drinking. The famous English author Iris Murdoch, who suffered from Alzheimer's at an advanced age, experienced this. Her husband John Bayley describes this in the second part of his impressive memoirs, *Iris and her friends*:

> *Thou mettest with things dying. I with things newborn.* It happens to me nowadays to be haunted by Shakespeare's line, which suggest that the two states are not so very different. Sometimes Iris's resemblance to a three-year-old is so uncanny that I find myself expecting her to shrink to an appropriate size.

My own enactment of a parent's role is equally exact, involuntarily faithful. Sometimes when I give her supper with a spoon, Iris will eat creamed rice of baked beans with a sort of negligent greed, like a child pretending it doesn't really want them, is above such things as food. More often, she turns her head away, and yet when I proffer a spoonful, she opens, her mouth obediently at once, like a chick on the nest. Being fed is still a pleasure to her.

'Bed now?' I say hopefully, but she doesn't care for the idea, or for any other course of action. She sits, and when I smile at her, she smiles back as if she knows perfectly well what I have in mind.

(Bayley 2000)

In the last phase the patient will not even be able to walk, just sit, until at a certain point even that will no longer be possible.

When great gaps appear in the memory, the patient's general good sense and intellect will inevitably suffer in consequence. The line between memory and intelligence, when analyzed closely, is fairly artificial. No memory means no intellect, and vice versa – they both need each other, just as the master and his servant need each other. If we want to remember something we have experienced, we will have to 'file' it properly in our memory library, as we have said before, and bring it into association with earlier experiences. These are intellectual skills. On the other hand, if we need to find a solution to a particular problem we will have to consult our memories in order to see how we approached similar problems in the past. In short, therefore, memory and intelligence merge. People suffering from mild dementia will sooner or later be unable to solve even the simplest of problems. Jokes will also be beyond their understanding, because in order to comprehend them we have to be able to make quick and easy associations.

We must also be able to view things from two perspectives at the same time; that is, literally and figuratively.

The further the memory rolls back, the more the person's thinking comes to resemble that of a small child, and all that that entails.

A child of 12 might think: 'I wouldn't like it if someone ate my food, so that means that others would probably not like it if I ate theirs.' The person with dementia, however, can only think from his own perspective. Whilst he might be very bothered by the cries and grunts of fellow residents, he does not realize that they too might be bothered by the same behaviour in him. He is less and less able to follow 'logical' arguments, and his way of thinking reverts steadily back to the level of a child. Here is an example of the fact that his thinking is increasingly regressing to a childish level:

> *Nurse*: Do you have a husband?
> *Elderly person*: Yes.
> *Nurse*: What is his name?
> *Elderly person*: John.
> *Nurse*: Does John have a wife?
> *Elderly person*: No.
> *Elderly person*: I want to go home to my father and mother.
> *Nurse*: You are almost 90 years old now. How old would your father and mother be now?
> *Elderly person*: 50 or 60?
>
> (Verdult 1993)

Sometimes this primitive way of reasoning leads to funny remarks, like the following:

Elderly person: Can you take me home?
Nurse: I don't know where you live.
Elderly person: Neither do I, but I can show you the way.

The consequences of this roll-back memory process can be summarized as follows:

- loss of instrumental skills, such as making coffee, using the vacuum cleaner, driving

- memory loss in terms of later and earlier phase events (his own retirement, for instance)

- decreased social skills and behaviour norms (loss of decorum)

- word loss, diminishing vocabulary, worsening speech capacity (aphasia)

- disorientation towards people: inability to recognize partner and children

- dead people are 'resurrected' from the past

- diminished self-care abilities: dressing, washing, teeth brushing, toilet use

- personality change

- deterioration in intellectual functioning.

The two laws of dementia described in this chapter change the life of the person concerned completely and utterly. What does the person actually do? How does he see his own illness? These questions will form the core of the following chapter.

Scientific support
for the second law of dementia

We have known for the last few years that, in Alzheimer patients, self-care activities (washing, dressing, eating and toilet use, etc.) are lost in reverse order to the sequence in which they were learned (Reisberg 1986; Reisberg, Ferris and Franssen 1986). The Reisberg research group which discovered this also went on to establish that this so-called retrogenesis is equally true of human intellectual development as a whole; the dementia patient follows the same cognitive development stadia of a child (as described by the famous Swiss psychologist Piaget), but in the reverse order (Sclan *et al.* 1990).

In terms of the brain, too, the dementia patient returns to his origins. It has been established, for instance, that the myelin sheaths (the coating of the nerve axons), which are the last to develop in the total process of human growth, are the first to disappear in dementia patients (Braak and Braak 1996). Another interesting aspect is that the reduced EEG activity we see in dementia is in fact a reflection of the normal increase we see in growing children (Cioni, Biagioni and Cipollini 1992). Surprisingly, too (Franssen *et al.* 1997), we see a return of the infant-reflexes (that is, the searching, gripping and sucking reflexes) in dementia. A geriatric patient with severe dementia might, for example, also reach the point of refusing all food and drink, but if he were to be given a baby's bottle (which does not look like a baby's bottle!), he might be inclined to drink again; that is, whilst he no longer sees the cup of tea or the sandwich as food (and thus pushes it aside), his sucking reflex is well able to 'understand' the purpose of the rubber mouth-piece on the bottle.

In short, the old expression 'second childhood' (a long-forbidden term) contains more truth than we (the experts) have been willing to believe for a very long time.

3

The experience of dementia

Introduction

A man remembers his grandfather thus:

> He had become completely child-like in the last few years. Very naughty. He shouted at Granny, left his food uneaten, complained about his children leaving home, and walked out of the house – these were probably all the things he had always wanted to do, and which his common sense now no longer prevented him from doing.
>
> He always had a stick with him when he walked along the dyke, and from time to time he pointed it in the direction of the sky. 'Pang,' he would say, 'there goes another one.' But no one knew what he meant by it.
>
> Atje came by sometimes and would say teasingly, as everyone did there: 'God, Jan, I have shot so many on my way here today.'
>
> Granddad was quick to respond with: 'Oh no, you can't kid me – there aren't any more left up there.'
>
> I once stood with him behind the house as we looked across the polder, and we saw a car passing in the distance.

'Look,' he said, 'a car' – but it had already disappeared
well beyond the horizon. He had a twinkle in his eye. You
felt that behind his mask, he knew exactly what was
going on. Sad really.

I have believed ever since that crazy people are the
same as everyone else, only worse.

(Van Zomeren 1987)

What is going on in my dear husband's head? What is he
thinking, what is he feeling? It is possible to give a reasonable,
although never complete, answer to these questions, so long as
he is functioning well and is mentally fit. As soon as someone
begins to go downhill, however, these questions become
unsolvable puzzles. We will have to develop dementia ourselves if we are ever to know what someone in the early stages
of dementia might be feeling, just as we will have to be dead
before we know what comes after it. In short, therefore, there
will never be a definitive answer to these questions.

Despite these limitations, however, this chapter will nonetheless attempt to sketch a picture of how someone might
experience his own dementing process. It is important that we
have some awareness of what dementia is in practice, because –
often without realizing it – we are quick to 'tune' our approach
to the dementia patient on what we see before us. If we think,
for instance, that he can control his anger, we will obviously
react differently towards him to how we would behave if we
had reason to believe that he might not be able to control
himself.

How can we know how someone is experiencing dementia?

There are three sources which provide us with a reasonable
picture of the dementia patient's 'world' and how he is experi-

encing it. The first source is what he conveys to us, in either the spoken or the written word. A good example of this is Van Delft's (1993) book *We komen niet meer waar we geweest zijn* (*We no longer go where we have been before*), in which she describes her talks with dementia patients.

The second source lies in the dementia patient's own behaviour. We can deduce, to a certain extent at least, how he is feeling, or what he is experiencing, on the basis of his tears or his laughter, his agitation or his calm, his aggression or his easy manner.

The third source is our own capacity to imagine or place ourselves in his shoes. Everyone loses track of things and knows how that feels, everyone is familiar with the twilight state that hovers between sleep and wakefulness, and everyone has woken up to the shock of finding themselves in a strange bed (realizing a few moments later that they are in a hotel). And that is how someone with dementia might feel too. Writers and poets are especially able to tell us what is going on in the head of a loved one suffering from dementia and in the heads of those around him. A fitting example of this is Bernlef's (1988) novel *Out of mind*.

Our ability to imagine can also be stimulated by the personal experiences which those who have suffered severe memory loss, without there being any question of dementia, have told us. Take the Russian soldier Zasetski, for instance, who sustained a bullet shot to his head during the Second World War, and then spent 25 years writing his thoughts in detail in his diary:

> I'm in a kind of fog all the times, like a heavy half-sleep. My memory's a blank. I can't think of a single word. All that flashes through my mind are some images, hazy visions that suddenly appear and just as suddenly

disappear, giving way to fresh images. But I simply can't understand or remember what these mean.

Whatever I do remember is scattered, broken down into disconnected bits and pieces. That's why I react so abnormally to every word and idea, every attempt to understand the meaning of words.

(Zasetski in Luria 1992)

The preliminary phase

In Gabriel Marquez's famous novel *Love in the time of cholera* one of the main characters, the aged doctor Juvinal Urbino, experiences the fear one can have in the preliminary phase of dementia.

> He stared at a blushing boy who nodded to him in greeting. He had seen him somewhere, no doubt about that, but he could not remember where. This often happened to him, above all with people's names, even those he knew well, or with a melody from other times, and it caused him such dreadful anguish that one night he would have preferred to die rather than endure it until dawn.

(Marquez 1988)

The same experience is described by the Spanish film maker, and 'the father of cinematic surrealism', Luis Buñuel in his memoirs:

> I'm overwhelmed by anxiety when I can't remember a recent event, or the name of someone I've met during the last few months, or the name of a familiar object. I feel as if my whole personality has suddenly disintegrated; I become obsessed; I can't think about anything else; and

yet all my efforts and my rage get me nowhere. Am I going to disappear altogether? The obligation to find a metaphor to describe 'table' is a monstrous feeling, but I console myself with the fact that there is something even worse – to be alive and yet not recognize yourself, not know anymore who you are.

You have to begin to lose your memory, if only in bits and pieces, to realize that memory is what makes our lives. Life without memory is no life at all, just as an intelligence without the possibility of expression is not really an intelligence. Our memory is our coherence, our reason, our feeling, even our action. Without it, we are nothing.

(Buñuel 2003)

Dementia begins with forgetfulness and increasingly not knowing things such as: what the time is; who called yesterday; where the door key is; what question has just been asked; or what the plans were for this morning, etc. Carrying out fairly complicated tasks according to sequence, such as cooking, repairing a bike and organizing a birthday party, demands tremendous effort on the part of someone with dementia. There will inevitably be some mishaps here and there. The frustration this causes will be expressed in annoyance on one occasion, and in despondency on another. There are also, however, moments of deep anxiety: fear of decline, fear of drifting into dementia. The anxiety storm lulls, however, as soon as the person concerned successfully busies himself with something else. 'Perhaps it's my age,' he might say.

The need-for-supervision phase

We can actually only speak of dementia if the brain disorder disrupts the individual's life so seriously that he is no longer able to cope without the help and support of others. This is the case when forgetfulness becomes more the rule than the exception. It is the phase in which frequent mishaps bring him into conflict with those around him, especially his partner or someone else sharing his home. It is also the phase in which he will become extremely adept at applying a rich stock of escape tricks, excuses and untruths, as well as kidding himself and others that things are not as bad as they might seem – to the extent, even, of claiming that 'all is well in the State of Denmark'. He attempts to sustain the image for those outside that the façade of the house is still intact, while in fact, total chaos reigns. Such attempts often add fuel to the fire: those around him frequently respond with frustration and anger.

Is the person with dementia aware of the decline?

The question people in his immediate environment find the most intriguing is: does the patient himself know what is happening to him? Studies carried out among people who have suffered a dramatic life event and have been left, in consequence, with a psychotrauma have taught us that the human spirit is capable of creating a protective barrier against insights that are too painful to contemplate. Our brains slam the door of knowledge shut when severe anxiety and total helplessness threaten to engulf us. In some cases, the door will remain hermetically sealed, although most people will manage to keep it open just a fraction, for shorter or longer periods of time. At these moments, we might hear them say such things as: 'My head feels empty', 'This is not me', or 'I can feel something is very wrong with me.'

The daughter of a mother with dementia considers this question of self-awareness:

She must realize. If you forget things so often, and lose track of what is going on today, then you must surely notice it? Mum, who in a moment of fury, climbed into her coat and announced to Dad: 'I don't need this any more. I might as well jump into the canal.' And by the time she reached the corner of the street, she had already forgotten what she had in mind. Was it a moment of intense unhappiness at what had overcome her? A real awareness of what was going on? Or did she feel betrayed by us, once again? We claimed that we had said and done certain things which she was no longer able to remember. In her eyes, everyone was lying. Everyone was trying to make a fool of her. Was it because of that?

We couldn't talk about it, but she did try to explain to me what she saw during her anxiety attacks.

'Then I look out of the window, and everything turns black. Everything seems to be disappearing into a vague hole – as if the space was being sucked in,' she gestured towards the window. And then she shook her head.

'No, it's more like an invisible roller-blind coming down.'

(Van den Berg 1995)

The memory of my father's last years that had made the deepest impression on me is described in the following:

When my father, as a result of Parkinson's disease and dementia combined, was able to undertake less and less, I regularly took him out for a drive in my car. We drove through the area where he had lived for the first 30 years of his life. He enjoyed seeing (and recognizing) the houses, streets, trees, and earlier landscapes again. On one of our drives through the area he had known so well, however, my father was clearly very troubled. It seemed as if he was imprisoned in himself. I wanted to know what was happening, and asked him 'Dad, what do you want?' His reply was so immediate and so loud that it shook the windows of my car: '*To live!*'

Not everyone is unhappy

Some people are so laid-back by nature for their entire lives that nothing and no one will ever throw them off course. Not even in the event of serious forgetfulness and mental decline.

We were totally content together; two happy people. Both of us. All the time. We were also quite content with everything that had happened to us. We ate an orange together, or…a biscuit. We enjoyed a…very small…drink together. And that was enough. We had no need for more, or for anything else. Neither of us felt any need for that. We enjoyed other things together. And that has not changed. That has never been interrupted by anything or anyone. The situation has remained exactly the same, as it always has been. Strange really.

I am a happy person. Yes. And I have enjoyed things as they are. Loesje [his deceased wife] says: 'Hansje is perfectly satisfied with this or with that. Hansje is always satisfied with what he has.' And that is true. I am a perfectly happy person. I can't explain it any other way. My overriding thought has been that I have never been discontented with my life. I put a high value on life. And have lived it accordingly. Really. I took the best from whatever crossed my path. What I did not like, I abandoned. I simply threw it away! I didn't want to have anything to do with it. So that's how it was.

(A man with dementia, quoted in Van Delft 1993)

If such people find themselves having to walk the road of dementia, they still manage to do so with their old air of contentment. They have always been happy and they are happy now, particularly if the atmosphere around them is warm and pleasing to them. Some even seem to be happier than ever; after all, many of life's worries and responsibilities have now fallen away.

It may be that some are happy for another reason. We have always assumed, until now, that people with dementia – albeit for just one fleeting moment – will know what is happening to them. It is quite possible, however, that the pieces of the memory melt away so slowly that the person concerned is totally unaware of it. In this case, the old saying 'Ignorance is bliss' fits such a person well.

Intensified personal characteristics

In the case of Alzheimer's, the literature mentions personality change. I often argued with Iris about the question of whether that was the case with her mother too. At first sight you would think it was. She became nicer and more affectionate, and increasingly thankful for little gestures, easier to get along with.

The sharp edges, all those dangerous projections on which you could badly hurt yourself, were ground by those last accelerations. In the mists of her old age she took on childish contours. Who could have predicted that some ten years ago…well, he or she did not know her.

At the same time she was still unmistakably herself. At her core there had always been great willpower and cleverness, and that was still there. You could even say that she only went more to the core in that respect. It went too far to suggest that all her sweetness was a deception, there

was no indication whatsoever to think she would be able
to evaluate her condition so effectively. But it was a fact
that she benefited from it. Everything became less,
everything except her ability to win people over.

   She was polite, she said 'please' and 'thank you'. She
was respectable. She crossed her legs as she was put in a
wheelchair. She was funny. She took every opportunity to
poke fun at herself and others. Her voice grew weaker, her
jokes stronger.

   Everyone loved her.

(Van Zomeren 2001)

People affected by dementia do not usually change completely.
Contented people usually stay content, and unhappy people
remain unhappy; most, however, hover somewhere between
the two. Just as with people without dementia, dementia
patients can be happy one moment, sad the next, only to be
followed a little later by fear and anger. The basic mood
remains in people with dementia much the same as it was
before. Certain personality traits, however, can become more
accentuated. Someone who is innately mistrustful by nature
can become even more mistrustful, and a kind and thoughtful
person can sometimes become even kinder and even more
thoughtful. It seems as if the pre-dementia personality
characteristics become more intense, although this need not be
so in all cases. Some personalities can change completely,
however: a pleasant and easy-going person can turn into a real
'misery-guts', tyrannizing everyone around him. The reverse is
also possible, and the 'misery-guts' can become the 'life and
soul of the party'.

   A daughter describes a change in her mother, and her own
response to it:

My mother and I are not exactly good friends. We have never been friends really. Not that we have frequent rows – strangely enough, we have never exchanged many words. Perhaps she felt there was no point in getting into an argument with me. Even as a child, I had the feeling that my mother was not really very fond of me. That feeling has increased through the years. My mother was, and is, only interested in herself. When I married, she was jealous of my simple pleasure in being happily married, in having a close and 'warm' family, and in having a job I thoroughly enjoyed. Now that she is less 'distant' and disapproving, I still find it difficult to like her. I feel like screaming at her: 'You are only doing it because you need me, because your three daughters-in-law have already given up on you. Your illness has changed you. And any feelings of regret or love have absolutely nothing to do with it.'

How someone experiences his illness is not only determined by what the illness does to him, but also by what he does with his illness. The way someone responds to the dementia, and the way in which he perceives it, depends on his personality, on what he has experienced earlier in his life, and on the way he acted and reacted in response to earlier problematical events in his life. If someone has always tended to be thrown quickly off balance, then he will also perceive his dementia as a disaster. If, on the other hand, someone is used to tackling problems head-on, and looking for solutions, then he will probably see his dementia from a less negative viewpoint.

It also has to be said that the way in which those in the patient's immediate vicinity react to the illness and its victim can determine how the sickness is experienced, just as much as the sickness itself.

Feelings dominate the thinking

Not only does the memory deteriorate, but the power to think as well. The person concerned is less able to reflect intellectually on things, his own behaviour included. In the case of people without dementia, there is usually a period of thought between feeling and action. If we are suddenly hit in the face by someone unknown to us, most of us will, first of all, try to gather our thoughts for a moment, in order to decide what to do in the circumstances: hit back, shout, escape, ask for an explanation, etc. This moment of reflection ensures that we do not automatically succumb to the first, and often intense, impulse that rises in us. Pondering for a moment usually results in a somewhat milder response.

The assault on the mental capacities, however, means that someone with dementia is more likely to be more impulsive and vehement in his responses. He is not deterred by such questions as: 'Can I really say that?', or 'Can I get away with this?' Impulse is his spur, and if he subsequently realizes what he has done he will probably be quite shocked.

In the course of this phase, the person with dementia will experience the so-called basic feelings only: disgust, sadness, anxiety, pleasure and trust. Any feelings that call for careful, premeditated thought disappear. Shame or regret imply knowledge of prevailing standards and, in order to show admiration and gratitude, we need to comprehend what someone's achievement has entailed.

The person with dementia also has no more feelings relating to either the past or the future. How can he foster hope, if the future no longer exists for him? How can he feel revenge if he cannot remember what another did to him? And how can he feel guilt or remorse about something he has long forgotten?

It is in this phase, therefore, that the person with dementia loses all contact with feelings such as shame, gratitude, guilt, hope, revenge and remorse.

A son said about his mother:

> It was not that she was forgetting discrete events; she was unable to place herself in a meaningful sequence of those events. She knew who she once had been, but not who she had become. Her memories of childhood were intact, but her short-term recollection had collapsed, so that past and present were marooned far from each other.

> (Ignatieff 1993)

The need-for-care phase

A letter from a lady with dementia in a nursing home read as follows:

Sunday

Beloved parents,

Although I cannot see as well as I used to, I will still try to write to you. How are you both? I hope you are both well. This is my first letter since I arrived here. There is *nothing* wrong with me. And I would very much like to leave this place and come to you. There is nothing wrong with me, only my eyes. I need a new pair of glasses, but unfortunately I do not have enough money. I hope you are both doing well. A visit is not possible. No one ever visits me. Only Suzy. There is nothing wrong with me. I

---

could easily go home. Anthony is also here but never visits me. He lives upstairs, I don't. I need some new glasses but have no money. May I come home please. Or have you written me off as your daughter. I have shed many tears of homesickness here. I have not had any post or suchlike since I came here. There are also very few visits. Only Suzy – she is a very faithful visitor. You have no idea how many tears I have shed here. The sister says there is absolutely nothing wrong with me. Imagine. All it costs is money and tears. The sister asked me only yesterday whether I had no family at all.

I will close now because my eyesight is so bad.

Warm greetings from your daughter.

Dot

In the previous phase, the person with dementia was no longer able to absorb any new information, because the 'recording' switch on the memory's video recorder had broken down. The 'play' switch was still working, however, and it meant that what the dementia patient had recorded prior to the start of his illness could still be viewed. In the course of the need-for-care phase, however, even the earlier video recordings show signs of serious wear and tear.

Back to the past

The monster of the roll-back memory results in the person concerned sinking back further and further into his recollections of the past; it also means that what he experiences is governed by themes which were important to him earlier in his life. The retired farmer will want to go to his cows several times a day, because they have to be milked. Every time someone tries to stop him doing this, he becomes distraught, angry or grieved. The same is true of the housewife who wonders desperately when her children will be coming home from school, and the geriatric patient with dementia who is deluded into thinking he is a child again and misses his parents.

Getting lost in time and space

The patient with dementia loses his sense of orientation in space and time, and repeatedly asks the questions: 'Where am I?', and 'What am I doing?' And if these questions are answered they often constitute insurmountable problems for him. He is lost, as it were.

> I still live with my father. Yes indeed, I was up early this morning. I-live-in-this-building...? HAHAHA. Surely not. That's not possible. I've lost my way completely. HAHAHA...no fooling. I don't know anything about it. But my parents do???
>
> My parents have...died...? I'm surprised. I don't understand. I was at home only last week. I had to collect something. That's strange. I can't imagine. No, that's not right. My father is not dead. He is still alive. Yes, I know that for certain! I hope so anyway. I would prefer that. I'll ask my mother some time. She's much more au fait than Pa.
>
> (A female dementia patient, quoted in Van Delft 1993)

When the familiar set contours of space and time fall away, the gulf between the world of people without dementia and the new, other world of the dementia patient becomes so large it cannot be bridged.

The more the dementia advances, the more difficult it becomes for the patient to think about who he is and what he is doing. The capacity to think about one's own emotions and behaviour calls for a considerable degree of thought-processing. If a person with dementia fails in some way, or is not successful at something, this has a very different meaning for him at this stage of his life than it would have done before the onset of the dementia. He might have thought then: 'I'm going wrong – I should have done this – and it means that I am going into decline', or 'I'm making mistakes – what will others think of me?' He is not able anymore to take on this kind of complex analysis. His thinking brings him no further now than: 'What I want is not happening.'

The mistakes no longer have any consequences for his self-image. His own identity has crumbled into so many pieces that it hardly exists any more. Disappointment and annoyance in the face of his own failures gradually disappear into nothing, and sometimes it seems – albeit briefly – that they have been replaced by mild surprise.

In the last period of the need-for-care phase, people with dementia simply allow events to roll over them like water off a duck's back, rather than take any kind of initiative. They simply wait and react when 'pricked'. Whilst a patient in an earlier phase would probably have taken steps to confront his 'opponent' after a disagreement, he now does nothing.

Most give the impression of no longer being actively interested in what the cause of their mistakes might be, but rather more in the question of how, and to whom, they can turn for help.

Painful past experiences rise to the surface

Many older people have experienced one or more dramatic events in their lives, such as an accident or a near miss; an attack; rape; physical and/or mental abuse; the violent death of a loved one; abandonment; death of a child; war experiences.

Dementia brings to an end a person's most tried and trusted way of confronting setbacks. The psychological 'dykes' which protect us against the floods of profound sorrow and despair also break down at this stage. It is for this reason that old psychological wounds can suddenly break open again on the surface. A life event today can evoke a life event from the past. That dreadful event *then* is suddenly relived as if it were taking place *now*. A door that is blocked can suddenly revive memories in the mind of someone with dementia of when he was held captive in a locked room with all the intense anxiety that that caused. Being held tightly by the wrist might remind a person with dementia that this was often the start of being mistreated by his father. The eyes or posture of a young woman might bring back to mind the moment when, as Holland was being liberated, a retreating German soldier suddenly killed a young woman right in front of the patient's eyes.

Someone with dementia may suddenly find himself, in broad daylight, going through a terrible nightmare, but it is not a dream for him – it is reality. Desperately frightened, like a wounded animal or an animal in great peril, he will lose control as he is unexpectedly confronted by the ghastly event of so many years ago. Emotions – if they have not been sufficiently worked through – retain their power. Emotional explosions, therefore, can reflect the 'breaking open' of old psychological wounds.

And then all kinds of long-suppressed anxieties from the past come unexpectedly to the surface in this process.

When World War II broke out, Justus was a reserve officer. Those days in May became for him and his infantry unit a short and unequal battle in Zeeland. Justus was confronted by the loss of several brave comrades, with the capitulation, with a humiliating retreat, and with the return to what was referred to as 'normal life', but which for the next five years would never be normal.

Tonight is different. I feel it. I follow him to the corridor. He is not looking for anything, but is peering anxiously into the semi-darkness. Something invisible spurs him into action. When he sees me, he grabs my arm and shouts: 'Duck!' In my ignorance I stand still, and he then puts his arm around my waist, opens the door of the toilet, and pushes me inside. He then shrieks: 'Look for cover. They are shooting!' With both hands, he pulls the door handle towards him, and with shaking fingers he tries to turn the knob to 'occupied'. In that limited space, he stands like a block before me. I feel the sharp edge of the sink pressing into my back. Tired and sleepy as I am, I can't really enter into this Wild-West scenario, and I say to him as I try to open the door: 'Go easy now chum, there's nothing going on. Come on.' Again he grabs me, and as I try to free myself, I am momentarily surprised by the power of his grip.

'Don't be stupid,' – again that sharp and anxious voice – 'if they shoot you dead, it's your own fault.' And there we stand. He with his bare feet on the round mat – I on the cold tiles.

(Prins 1997)

Confidence in the other

The more the dementia relentlessly advances, the more sensitive the patient becomes to how others relate to him. Because he is less and less able to understand what is being said to him, he will become more and more susceptible to body language, facial expressions, gestures and tones of voice. The way in which the dementia patient will judge those around him is to a certain extent comparable to the way we ourselves form judgements about people we can hear but cannot see. Rather like a television programme with the sound turned off.

That the person with dementia is more aware of the non-verbal aspects of communication is not only a question of his no longer being able to understand the content of a conversation as well as he would have done before his illness. A second reason is that his relationship with those around him has now also become much more important for him. To survive, he *needs* the help of others. It is absolutely essential for him to 'feel' that those around him can be trusted and that they mean well towards him. In these terms, he becomes more and more like a small child who, in order for his needs to be satisfied, is largely reliant on others. If the dementia patient feels able to place his trust in his carers, he will feel at ease, but if that trust is missing he will become anxious.

The patient's perception of things is disturbed

'Don't you see?' my brother said. 'She has forgotten the grammar of the cinema, how you go somewhere and sit in the dark and watch the golden girl growing larger and larger, all seen from the eye of God. No wonder she was frightened.'

'But,' I said, 'she remembered the chalice with the palace.'

'Because she remembers where she was and who she was with,' my brother said. 'What she can't remember is her relation to new images. She can't say, I am here in my seat, and this is just a film. It took her over completely.'

I remembered how my wife and I used to take our kids to the movies when they were small, and how when they saw a wolf bound across the screen at them, they shrieked and buried their heads in our laps. I could remember envying our children and thinking how diminished it was to be in control of the process of illusion.

Illness had returned my mother to the condition of my children. There was no distance, no membrane of knowing between her and the screen. She was, like them, defenceless before the wolf.

'What happened in the movie might be what is happening to her memory images,' my brother said. 'She sits in the movie theatre of her own mind and she doesn't know what these images are or what her relation to them is supposed to be. There's just one damned thing after another.'

I was thinking how crazy it must seem not to possess your own memories any more: the fire in the back pasture, and voices calling and the smell of cinders and a man in bathing trunks with a hose, none of it making sense because it no longer belonged to you, because you couldn't understand why these images were scrabbling across the white screen of your mind.

(Ignatieff 1993)

The dementia patient's senses pick up information in much the same way as they have always done. The more he deteriorates mentally, however, the less able he will be to process that information. He will have to resort more often to asking those around him what he is seeing or hearing. Asking questions, however, does not help – because the answers he is given are often too difficult. The ability to 'file' information in his head and remember it has now gone forever. The information still flows in his direction, but he cannot absorb it.

The more difficult it becomes to process information, the more he will 'retreat' from those around him and take refuge in himself. He will sit with eyes closed, for increasingly larger parts of every day: drowsing and sleeping.

The need-for-nursing-care phase
In search of safety and trust

A daughter contemplates her mother's memory loss thus:

> Whilst her memory was once a kind of worm-eaten apple, there is practically nothing left of it at all now. The expression is inward-looking. She peers into an empty space. And for some time now, she has not seen anything passing outside. There is no more future. Her children are now in charge of her memory. It is we who have to remember her past, and thus our own childhood pasts. We have to remember now who was already walking at thirteen months, and who used to gather pieces of spinach between cheeks and gums and suddenly spit them out in a big arc. She will no longer talk about who said 'weeny bite' when he saw her mouth chewing and wanted something, and about who nearly died from German measles.
>
> (Hilhorst 1999)

In the last phase of his journey towards his own sunset – as the former American President Ronald Reagan commented when informing the world of his own dementing process – someone with dementia is hardly able to act with any purpose or proper coordination. He no longer goes in search of stimuli – indeed, he cannot. Perhaps his experience of the things around him, in this phase of his life, is the same as that of the infant. Like a small child – vulnerable and dependent on others – the patient's life at this stage revolves around the satisfaction of his most primary physical needs, eating, drinking, rest and warmth, and of his emotional needs too, in the form of safety and trust.

Every communicative sign he makes, such as physical restlessness, cries of panic, the call for contact and sobbing, are all directed to satisfying these needs in him. It may be that, because he no longer recognizes people around him, he experiences the same anxiety as a child missing its mother; the sunken body, like that of an unborn baby in the womb, is perhaps the physical expression of this.

A nurse's description of this phase is as follows:

> Four years ago I worked in a nursing home, where I took care of a lady with severe dementia who lay in bed all day in a foetal position and with her cuddly toy in her arms. Verbal communication was no longer possible. With soft sounds, and sometimes with some eye contact and touching, she could still be reached. She loved these moments.
>
> When one morning I looked into her room, I heard her crying softly. Because she could no longer say what was wrong, I whispered sweet words to her, stroked her hair and moved her. Then I gave her a drink, but nothing worked. She kept crying. I moved her again and shook

her pillow, but again without result. Big tears now ran down her cheeks.

Spontaneously I lowered the bed frame on the side, lay down beside her on the blanket and held her in my arms. Immediately she lay her head on my shoulder, babbling, put her hand in my sleeve, stroked my upper arm and said 'Mama, Mama' a couple of times. I felt the tension flow out of her body. She fell asleep in my arms. Very carefully I moved her back onto her pillow and got out of the bed. So that was it: she was missing her mother, her sense of security.

Three weeks later she died.

Nature has, fortunately, found a very good medicine to counteract such a degree of anxiety: an insatiable need for sleep. Because the past and the present have both been wiped completely from his memory, he no longer has any sense of time. He is living in an endless 'now'. Only what is happening in the here and now is real.

Decreased consciousness

The dementia patient's world actually consists of no more than his own body. He is barely able to understand anything of what is happening around him. The sound of cups and plates is no longer a sign for him that tea is on its way. He does not know any more that he is meant to drink from the mug standing on the table in front of him. Only when someone brings it to his mouth, and he feels the dampness on his lips, will he, in a kind of reflex action, begin to drink from it. Smell, touch and taste have now become more important senses than hearing and seeing. The limited behavioural signs he exhibits are primarily physical in nature. If he does not want certain food or a particular drink, he will make it clear by turning his head away, by pressing his lips tightly together, by gesturing his refusal, or by spitting the food or drink out of his mouth. Some patients refuse entirely to eat or drink in this phase – it is their way, perhaps, of signalling to us that they have had enough of it all.

In the final phase of his life, the dementia patient will only absorb information in a vaguely conscious way. His perception of things is reminiscent of anaesthesia or decreased consciousness in people without dementia. To all appearances, the distinction between the individual person and his environment has disappeared. He does not recognize himself any more. He sometimes looks at his feet and arms as if they were objects separate from himself. It could be that he regards his own body as strange and unfamiliar.

The very last to go in the whole dementing process is the capacity to smile. If he can no longer do that, then death is not far away.

4

Communication

Introduction

Two women with dementia who have both recently been
admitted to a nursing home are talking together:

> 'It is comfortable and pleasant here, but it's not the
> same as home.'
> 'I just want to go and see whether the boys are home.'
> 'We have had a fine time here. We can certainly
> recommend it.'
> 'I am happiest with my parents. But we mustn't
> complain, we should be happy with what we've got. Do
> you know whether my mother is here?'
> 'You will have to wait and see. Because we have been
> taken away from home, we just don't know what's going
> on any more.'
> 'The people here are very kind, but...'
> 'I am going to ask anyway if we can go home.
> Mothers always like to have their children around them.'
> 'My children are adults.'

'I don't know. What will happen to them now? We haven't got our own house.'

'I have my own house in Amsterdam. You have your own house too.'

'But I would still like to be with my mother again.'

'I want to go to Amsterdam – my parents live there too.'

'I want to go to Poland. I want to fly and run home, preferably to my father. My grandmother is still alive too.'

'I don't look ahead like that. It never works out the way you want.'

(Den Tex 1990)

It is through both the spoken and the written word that people are able to share their experiences, feelings, desires and ideas.

Communication gives us the feeling of being bonded to others. Dementia, on the other hand, means in practice that the capacity to share experiences with others gradually disappears. The dementia patient is less and less able to talk to others in the normal way. It takes so much more effort for him to explain clearly to others what it is he is feeling or needing. At the same time, it also costs him ever-increasing effort to understand what others are trying to make clear to him. In a normal conversation between two people, both contribute more or less equally to it. This balance is no longer present, however, when we try to converse with someone suffering from dementia. We have to invest much more energy into our endeavours to communicate effectively with a dementia patient. The more advanced the dementia, the more energy will be required to achieve any degree of real communication.

Communication in the three phases of dementia

In the first stage, the need-for-supervision phase, the dementia patient is no longer able to talk about recent events, and often has difficulty in finding the right words. In any kind of conversation, he will increasingly resort to words that are vague and unclear. Examples of these so-called 'empty words' are: 'it'; 'somewhere'; 'things'; 'something'; 'someone'; 'people'; 'so'; 'them'. These words are referred to as 'empty' because they give no indication of anything concrete – 'I can't find that thing, it must be somewhere', for instance.

If the dementia patient makes a mistake in naming an article, he will often choose a word that is 'close' to the correct one: 'pen' instead of 'pencil', for example. In most cases, however, dementia patients in this phase understand quite well what is being said to them.

In the middle, need-for-care, phase the person with dementia will find it more and more difficult to engage in conversation of any kind, and will usually do so far less frequently than was his custom in the past. For those around him, it becomes quite a task to understand him, because he takes it for granted that they will automatically know what he is talking about. There are no introductory words or sentences which would normally lead the listener into the conversation – our patient simply starts his conversation from somewhere in the middle, and he cannot, of course, see the situation from the perspective of his listener.

He can no longer grasp the meaning of abstractions such as 'intelligence', 'politics', 'idea' or 'chance'. There is also no difference, in his mind, between the present situation and the past. The chair in the lounge of the nursing home does not *remind* him of a chair he might have had earlier in his life – the chair he sees now *is* that chair from the past. It is his own chair.

Linguists would see this as an example of there being no distinction between the sign and the object (Pols 1992).

It is also impossible for our patient to relate a well-constructed and logical story; the 'feed-back' process which links what we have said to what we are going to say is now beyond his capabilities, and it means that conversations have no beginning and no end. The 'conversation' quoted at the beginning of this chapter is a good example of this.

It costs someone with dementia tremendous effort to put a good sentence together and in order to cope as best he can he, quite understandably, retreats into a series of automatisms and standard phrases.

> He talks less and less these days. We haven't really had a proper conversation for a long time now, and even the most simple and ordinary conversation is difficult now... You can see Justus wrestling with his decimated vocabulary. He is hardly able to put the letters he has struggled so hard to find into words, and complete sentences demand too much of him now. He has, nonetheless, found a method of camouflage in this too. He has, for instance, a stock of standard sentences at hand, which on first hearing might sound quite normal, and he uses them with considerable skill.
>
> When Paul [a neighbour and friend] makes one of his frequent visits, he is given a friendly greeting and immediately asked: 'And, how was your holiday?' Now that holidays are no longer restricted to one period of the year only, this kind of question can be utilized all year round. Remarks such as: 'Have you had a good day?', 'It was nice of you to come', and 'What's the weather like today?', have become set items in his self-constructed vocabulary. And he can respond to any comment with a standard: 'Yes, that's the way it goes these days.'

A more lengthy visit opens with one of his standard sentences presented with suitable verve, after which – as he quickly loses the thread of what is being said – he withdraws into silence.

(Prins 1997)

In the last phase of dementia, the need-for-nursing-care phase, the patient will have completely lost his ability to talk; he cannot even produce the most 'ritual' of sentences. His verbal capacities are all but entirely gone, apart from some unarticulated noises. He is hardly able to respond to any kind of question, and reacts only to physical impulses such as pain, warmth, cold or movement (Pols 1992).

As has already been stated in the introduction to this chapter, the patient's capacity to communicate fades away step by step. In the next chapter, we will endeavour, nonetheless, to present some general tips and useful advice on how to communicate with someone with dementia as effectively as possible.

Basic attitude

It is very important to ensure that a conversation with a relative/partner/patient who has dementia does not have to compete with penetrating background noises, such as a loud radio or television. This demands extra effort on the patient's part to concentrate on what is being said.

We, the carers, must also ensure that we ourselves are not under any kind of time pressure, for instance. The potential for successful communication is at its highest when we are able to focus exclusively on the person with dementia and his specific needs. Do everything possible, too, to avoid whispering in his presence.

A daughter, wiser now, having learned the hard way, said:

If I am speaking with someone in mother's presence it is better to talk loudly, because if I whisper she becomes suspicious. I have to bear this particularly in mind when I am talking on the phone to someone.

In terms of respect, it is also important to remember that we should never talk about someone with dementia (in his presence) in the third person; that is, never say 'the patient is looking well today'.

Verbal communication

Keep communication simple and straightforward. 'It is three o'clock, time for a drink. Would you like tea or milk?' Someone with dementia will lose track of long and complicated announcements. The same is true if he is presented with two or more possibilities, such as: 'Shall we have a cup of tea and then go for a short drive?'

Requests to do something are best made immediately before they are due to take place. Never say, for instance, 'Would you like to…in five minutes' time?', or 'Shall we…later?', but rather 'Would you like to…now?'

It is wise to ask the question 'Would you like to…?' in the area or situation in which you want it to take place; for example, requests to get dressed should be voiced in the bathroom or the bedroom, and questions about what to eat or drink in the kitchen.

Make a habit of checking whether or not the person with dementia has actually understood what has been said. A simple 'yes' or 'no' is not always sufficient. Make sure he really does what you have asked – taken his pills, for instance. If he does something else in response to the question, then he has probably not understood it. It may be, however, that he did understand the question, but would not, or could not, respond to it.

One of the effects of dementia is that the brain needs much more time to process the information feeding into it. Someone with even mild dementia, for instance, will soon require five times more information-processing time than people unburdened by the disease.

> If someone asks him a question, it might take some time for him to formulate an answer that, not infrequently, will only in very broad terms have anything to do with the question asked. In the course of time, I have developed a kind of decoding system, but outsiders still engaged in the conversation might have difficulty in reconciling the answer with the question, and then find themselves nodding politely or simply shrugging it off with a bland 'yes'.
>
> (Prins 1997)

The best explanation is usually 'let's see what you mean'. Demonstrating what you want is the often most effective means of communication: the risks of misunderstandings are thus reduced to a minimum. A step beyond demonstrating what you want is to help the person with dementia to make the first move, such as giving him a towel and then 'steering' his hand in the direction of drying his arms or legs.

For family members or carers, one of the most difficult aspects of dealing with early-phase dementia is the tiring, non-productive, 'yes I did/no you didn't' kind of discussion. There is a tendency for the carer to want to put the patient 'right' if he says something that is not true, and before they know it they find themselves embroiled in a battle in which there are only losers. Two of the most important guidelines to remember in such situations, are therefore:

1.   Try to avoid 'yes/no' discussions as much as possible.

2.   Do not allow yourself to get upset about things that really do not matter: whether or not, for instance, a certain question has already been asked, or whether it is Tuesday or Wednesday today.

In order to be able to sail successfully on the current of what the other insists is right, we need to accept that the 'other' is suffering from dementia and is therefore almost in another world in another time. Resisting the hard truth of the situation means that from time to time you will inevitably find yourself at loggerheads with your patient.

> I believed for a long time that the truth was important. If my mother said it was April and it was in fact May, I felt I had to correct her immediately. A battle of words followed. And then at a certain moment, I thought: 'I'm mad, what does it matter if she thinks it's April?' That was a very liberating moment. And from that moment on, we had far fewer clashes and a much more pleasant contact.
>
> (A grandson)

There are moments and situations, of course, in which you *must* correct your patient or put him 'straight' on something: when he tries to put his right foot into his left shoe, for instance; but before intervening, consider for a moment how you prefer to be corrected. The answer would probably be: in as unobtrusive, calm and friendly a manner as possible. This is what the dementia patient wants, too. Get him back on the right track, therefore, by means of a gentle remark such as: 'It is really not important, but…', or 'Don't worry about it – we all make mistakes from time to time.'

It is possible to understand most behaviour of dementia patients – unwilling or non-cooperative type behaviour especially – if we realize that our patient also wants to avoid mistakes and hide his shortcomings, just as we do.

A daughter's account of her father illustrates this well:

> My father is mad about his two budgies. He watches them for hours on end. I have noticed recently, however, that he sometimes forgets to feed his beloved pets. And because Dad would be inconsolable if they died of hunger, I have tried to keep a watchful eye on things.
>
> When I noticed today that the bag of bird-feed I had bought yesterday had not been opened, I said: 'Dad, would you like to feed the budgies?' To my amazement, he replied: 'No, I don't feel like it right now.'
>
> When I had recovered from my surprise and given some thought to this unexpected retort, I got the feeling that he probably did not know where to look for our stocks of bird-feed any more. I decided, therefore, to rephrase the question half an hour later: 'Dad, I have bought a new bag of bird-feed for the budgies, and I have put it in the cupboard under the stairs. Perhaps you would like to give some to the budgies.' And at this point, he did get out of his chair, and within a few minutes was obviously enjoying the sight of the birds pecking away at the new food supply in their cage.

In order not to embarrass relatives/patients with dementia, it is better to avoid asking any questions about things that happened a short time ago. If you do decide, however, to start a conversation about something that had taken place earlier that day or week, then the best way to do it is to put it in the form of a confirmatory type of question, such as: 'John and little Sophie were here this afternoon, weren't they, Mum?'

Some relatives tend to bombard the patient with questions, usually during their visits to him in the nursing home. What they forget, however, is that he is also interested in their stories, especially when they concern people of whom he is particularly fond. It is important, therefore, to tell him what you have been doing; what has made you laugh; what has saddened you; the friends you have seen lately, etc. It does not matter if the patient does not completely comprehend what is being said; he will still enjoy the feelings and emotions that 'shine' out from your story, as well as the non-verbal messages contained in the intonation, the eyes, the facial expressions and the body language. Telling your story gives the dementia patient the feeling that he matters and that he belongs. The very fact that you are talking to him, and him alone, is more important by far than your actual words.

Non-verbal communication

Always try to speak in a calm and even tone – there is no need to raise your voice. Although most of us tend to speak more loudly to people who, for all sorts of reasons, are less able to understand what is being said, it is important not to do this. A person with dementia often interprets a loud voice as an angry voice, to which his response can be anger, sadness, restlessness or anxiety.

A superior tone and attitude, which places you 'above' someone with dementia, lessens considerably the chances of the message coming across as it should. A tone of voice which conveys a genuine sense of equality and friendliness is often the key to easy-going and smooth communication. A smile can also do wonders.

A grandchild made this observation:

My smile is my most important asset with my grandfather. When I smile at him, doors that normally stay closed suddenly fly open. And then everything is okay and I can do no wrong.

The general rule with dementia patients is to maintain eye contact as much as possible, and never to turn your body away from him. If you take steps to keep yourself within his field of vision when speaking to him, or when helping him in some way, you will find that he will interact more flexibly with you. Some people with dementia can become quite panicky when approached or spoken to from behind. Because they can no longer take the situation in at one glance, they can become anxious, which is then expressed in irritation and sometimes even in aggression. Explain what is happening, as far as possible. 'That's the door-bell, it will probably be Mrs Brown. She said she would come around this time.'

It is better to talk about matters which, at the same time, people with dementia can also hear, see, smell, feel or touch. A daughter expressed it as follows: 'You cannot take what they have always known as your starting point any more – you can only put trust in, and build on, what they are experiencing now.' This situation can be helped by the use of memory devices; that is, you point to things, or you show what you want to talk about. If you want to talk about the weather, for instance, position the person with dementia so that he has a good view of what is going on outside: by opening the curtains and by pointing to the rain, the clouds, the snow or the sun. Short but to the point, you might explain to someone a hundred times that it's spring, but it is perhaps only when you actually lay a lamb in his lap that he will really understand.

Insight into the past

Because memories of experiences in the distant past can be stored for much longer than those in a (more) recent phase of life, we advise linking conversations directly to the dementia patient's earlier customs, interests, preferences and experiences. You might, for instance, talk about his parents, his brothers and sisters, the happy moments of his youth, the primary school years, his work, 'calf love', his first really amorous adventures, and so on. It is, of course, better to draw him out on experiences of which you know he retains happy memories. Because the past often merges into the here and now, homing in on these early experiences is sometimes the only way of gaining contact with the dementia patient, and putting him at his ease.

A nurse here describes a successful technique she has used with one patient:

> I have known a man on our ward who earned his livelihood as a farmer. His wife told me that every week, for thirty years, he had gone to the market to sell one or two of his cows.
>
> When I came to work each morning, I always used to call on him to buy a few cows from him, and with a few hand-claps the deal was done. For him, it meant his day had been successful. He had the feeling that his work had been done, and for the rest of the day he was perfectly happy and satisfied.
>
> When this man was first admitted to my ward and he started to talk about his cows, a student nurse several times made the mistake of confronting him with the reality by telling him that he had not had a farm for the last ten years and that he had no more cattle. He was in total panic, and he remained anxious and restless for the rest of the day.

Focus on feelings

Memories of the past, and emotions generally, appear to suffer less from the break-down of the memory process in people with dementia. Perhaps it has something to do with the fact that feelings are timeless and therefore do not nestle in the memory where all kinds of information is kept, but that their roots go much deeper in fact.

A daughter expressed it as follows:

> My father is becoming more and more lonely. If a baby can experience feelings of loneliness, then a man with dementia can also feel terribly alone. He can also be happy and very content. Yes, just like a child.

One of the greatest challenges in gaining meaningful contact with people with dementia is to do everything possible to discover the sense behind the apparent non-sense, whereby the sense is often couched in a feeling or emotion.

If a relative with dementia is becoming anxious because she has to care for her children ('My children will be home from school soon'), who have actually lived independent lives for the last 25 years, you might say: 'Tell me something about your children – you are obviously missing them a lot.' What this mother is trying to say is that her children are constantly in her mind. Giving her the time and space to talk about her offspring, and her feelings for them, will help her to feel more 'at home' and on trusted ground, because her children have always been her pride and joy. By talking with her about them, she will feel she is being taken seriously. Another example: a patient with dementia announces that she is pregnant. Instead of reminding her of her age, you can respond to the expression on her face: 'I can see it on your face – you are obviously delighted.'

If you do not know immediately what the background feeling is, you might try to reflect the words or paraphrase them. If, for example, the patient refers to his fellow residents in the nursing home in terms of 'They are all off their rockers here', you could say: 'Oh, so you don't think they are quite in order then?' This often brings you a step further, and you discover that the patient feels neither 'at home' nor at ease in the nursing home.

When talking is no longer possible

Bearing in mind that the dementing process in the course of time will wipe out old information in the memory, a person with dementia will gradually feel increasingly helpless when people start to talk to him about earlier periods and past events in his life. When you notice that the dementing process has advanced this far, it is nonetheless still possible to sustain a worthwhile degree of contact and communication.

When words are no longer understood, your body can still 'speak' to your patient: you can put your arm around his shoulders, give him a gentle pat on his head, stroke his arm, hold his hand, smile at him. To the very end, a person with dementia will always be able to recognize the melody of a sentence or a phrase. Just as with babies and pets, someone with dementia can hear very well whether or not your words are friendly, unfriendly or sad, even though the meaning of the words, as such, no longer penetrate his understanding. Ultimately, you can communicate simply by 'being there'. The calm presence of someone he knows and trusts is tantamount to saying: 'Don't worry, I'm here, you're quite safe.' Patients with severe dementia will need this especially.

A daughter put it thus:

It is an illness that ultimately kills, an illness that blows all memories away. But once you have accepted that, you can still lead a happy life. It is a cliché, but the only thing that matters for her is that she is loved. If she feels that, then everything is okay. That feeling of love can be shared. And particularly so because she knows, far better than I, how to live in the here and now. The love she feels is not burdened, for instance, by the thought that potatoes have to be peeled.

5

Mood problems
Aggression, depressiveness and suspiciousness

Introduction

Dementia is often accompanied by emotional changes, and it is often very difficult for the family to understand and manage them. In this chapter we will cover three of the most frequently occurring mood problems: aggression, depressiveness and suspiciousness. We will discuss their possible causes and suggest ways of dealing with them. In order to be able to cope with troublesome behaviour of any kind, it usually helps to try to put yourself in the other's shoes. Before formulating the backgrounds and approach suggestions, we will undertake some thought-experiments, as a means of introducing the three mood problems. Understanding usually only develops by trying to empathize with the other, and by putting ourselves, as far as we can, in his situation.

Aggression

Imagine everything seems to be against you. You keep on making mistakes and messing things up. You lose things several times a day. You regularly find yourself unable to answer a question put to you. You are planning to do something, but only a few seconds later you discover that you have forgotten what you had in mind. Even the simple act of tying your shoe-laces or buttoning your shirt turns into a fiasco. Seldom, if at all, are you praised for what you have managed to achieve. No, instead of compliments, you are told in no uncertain terms every day what you have failed to do. Fortunately, you very quickly forget most of what is thrown at you, although it does leave you feeling rather damaged and unhappy. It only needs one more very small mishap, one more critical comment, and you are ready to hit the roof.

Ask yourself how you would feel if you were in this situation: Imagine you were one day suddenly transported to an unknown world. Everything looks strange around you, and you cannot make yourself understood in either the written or the spoken word. Suddenly, someone you do not know comes toward you and takes you by the hand. You have no idea what he wants from you. What would you do?

Causes

There is seldom just one explanation for human behaviour. There are usually several factors which 'steer' people in a particular direction. If we are asked about the motives behind our actions, however, we usually limit ourselves to one explanation only. To justify our actions, we usually resort to saying something that sounds fairly reasonable, such as: 'I was so busy – and that's why I flared up so quickly'; the other factors, therefore, lie hidden under the lid of our subconscious.

We discussed earlier the first explanation for aggressive behaviour in cases of dementia when we looked at the indirect consequences of disturbed encoding, namely frustration. We saw that aggression is a normal human reaction to a difficult situation, the instrument we use in our efforts to regain control of our lives.

The second explanation is that aggression can also be a reaction to sorrow, shame or some other, less fundamental, emotion. It demands much of the human soul to give full expression to such 'high' emotions. Even people not suffering from dementia often find it difficult to ventilate such feelings. Many of us feel angry when things appear to go against us. In the same way as children, we also show anger more readily than sorrow or shame. Out of the magic box of our emotions, we are only able to reveal the one closest to the surface – that is, anger. People hovering on the brink of dementia also do very much the same. Indeed, they cannot do otherwise.

The third explanation for aggression concerns the fact that, because of the less effective mental capacities which arise from the disorder, someone with dementia is less able to assess properly the situation he is in. He can no longer exercise his former intellectual capacity to understand the intentions of others. If someone reaches out the hand of friendship to him, he might see it – for instance – as the prelude to being slapped across the face, to which his response – naturally – is to hit out at the other, in an act of pure self-defence.

We have to go back to the individual's childhood to find the fourth explanation of aggression in dementia. Some children can be extremely volatile during the first 5 to 15 years of their lives. One word out of place, one small disappointment, one moment of seeming neglect can all give rise to acute anger. Only later in our lives do we learn to react differently.

Or as a doctor once explained to a dementia patient's daughter:

> One of the symptoms of this disease is called emotional incontinence. In most human beings there is an innate

tendency for going for what we want even if that means becoming aggressive with others. Parents bring us up not to behave in that way. What may be eroded in MID is the capacity to dampen down or repress these primitive feelings, as getting drunk causes us to forget to inhibit our desire to tell our best mate that we love him or strip down to our underpants in the middle of the high street. Let's face it, we've all been there.

(Quoted in Grant 1998)

As we grow up, however, we learn and discover that we can achieve much more if we remain calm and mature, rather than allow ourselves to react compulsively. We discover that people find us more likeable, and that we can be much more effective, if – when necessary – we subjugate our own feelings to those of the other. We come to the conclusion that the world does not revolve around us, and that we are merely one individual among billions of others. And finally, we learn to take account of others by getting to know them better. We learn, for instance, from the tone of voice, whether what is being said is meant to be taken seriously or as a joke. This handy and sensible manner of keeping the lid on impending aggression is taken from us in dementia. If we ask a patient with dementia to control his anger in the face of disappointment, we are actually asking too much of him.

Finally, we should remember that some people with dementia have been volatile and quick-tempered for most of their lives. Aggression in this case, therefore, constitutes no real break with the past: it is rather more an intensification of what was already there.

Prevention is better than cure

How should we deal with aggression in people with dementia? Before going more deeply into this facet, there are two things you must remember when someone is acting aggressively towards you: there must be *no discussion* and *no reprimand*. Both strategies are totally counterproductive.

Preventing aggressive outbursts is obviously the best tactic, but in order to do this we need to know the sources of the aggression. You can achieve this by carefully observing and registering what is making the person concerned so angry. The more methodical the registration, the easier it is to get to the root of the problem. A simple and very necessary aid in this is a notebook, with each page divided into five rows (see Table 5.1).

You use the first row, 'Time', to note the time of day the problem behaviour occurred – '7 a.m.', for instance. You indicate in the second row the situation or environment in which the aggression took place. Or, even better, you give a short description of the situation immediately *before* the incident. You write, for instance, 'in the bedroom' or 'in bed'. 'I tell her she has to get up and get dressed. I then take her by the arm and gently ease her into a sitting position.'

The third row indicates the particular problem you are trying to deal with. Here you might write 'foul language' or 'aggression'. (This row can also be used to denote other aspects of the condition, like depression, mistrust and other mood problems, as well as for behaviour problems such as wandering.)

The fourth row is there to give some indication of your own reactions to your patient's aggression. You might note, for instance, 'I tried with reasonable arguments to persuade him to dress himself', or 'the situation irritated me, and I pulled him sharply to his feet'.

In the last row, you give a short description of the result of the reaction; for example, 'he pulled the sheet over his head', or 'ugly words shouted in anger'.

When you have done this for approximately two weeks, it is very likely that you will see a certain behaviour pattern emerging. The aggression occurs, for instance, at the same time of the day, in the same situations, or your response to it is more or less the same every time.

Table 5.1 Methodological registration	
Time	07.30
Circumstances prior to the incident	In the bedroom: I tell Mary it's time to get up and get dressed. I try to get her onto her feet by gently pulling her by the arm.
Mary's reaction	Swearing
My own reaction	I try, using gentle persuasion, to encourage Mary to get up and dress herself.
Result of my reaction	Mary pulls the sheets over her head. She then throws verbal abuse at me.

If your partner/relative exhibits aggressive behaviour at the same time every day, it is worth experimenting with the situation. In Mary's case (see above), for instance, the carer could try to delay waking her until 8.30 a.m. – perhaps Mary is still just too sleepy at 7.30 a.m. and needs to sleep on for a while. Another possibility is to bring the waking hour forward. Recent research has shown that the biological clock of old people in the early stages of dementia differs from the norm. Getting up at 6 a.m., for instance (and going to bed earlier), might suit their bio-rhythm much better.

A second possibility is to change the situation, or put one's own stamp on it. Before waking Mary, for instance, the carer could open the curtains and turn the radio on softly – with the result that 15 minutes later, Mary might be much more receptive to being brought out of her slumber. Many people find it difficult to be woken abruptly – they need time to absorb the transition from night into day.

A third possibility is to react differently to the problem. Instead of entering into a discussion with Mary, or using reasonable arguments to persuade her, the carer might perhaps be able to break the deadlock by broaching a completely different subject, one which she knows Mary is interested in, and one which will quickly and willingly bring her out of her sleep.

The carer's attitude

Aggression in a dementia sufferer can also be provoked by the behaviour of the person most directly involved in his or her care. Just as a mother, by her attitude or tone of voice, can often provoke a very unpleasant tantrum in her baby or toddler, so too can the reaction of a partner or carer provoke tremendous frustration and annoyance in someone with dementia. We strongly recommend, therefore, that carers keep a very watchful eye on what kind of behaviour provokes the angry response. A word spoken too harshly; a hint of irritation in the carer's voice; an authoritative or patronizing way of speaking; a slightly aloof attitude; a mildly 'accusing' remark: things like these can all touch the raw nerves of someone with dementia and ignite the fire. If you ask a partner/relative with dementia to do something, he might feel he is being pushed or ordered against his will. You can, however, make the question sound more like a friendly suggestion which he/she is free to refuse. In this case, the person concerned is more likely to cooperate than when he is given no 'elbow room' in which to manoeuvre. A smile or a few friendly words (in which your request for cooperation is 'cloaked') can, in this case, often result in your not having to face a wall of resistance.

One of the best ways of calming an angry person is to take his anger seriously. You can do this by putting what he is feeling into words: 'I can see you are angry (with me).' Emotions need – primarily – to be acknowledged, and as soon as this is done the 'heat' usually drops.

Another possibility is that you do everything possible – seriously and calmly – to draw the person away from the source of his stress. Some people quieten down if you touch them, take them by the hand, or hug them. For others, on the other hand, you might have to be much more careful in using physical contact once the anger has 'kicked-in' – your patient might regard it as threatening, and thus his anger will only increase. In this case, therefore, keeping a reasonable distance and talking calmly is likely to be more effective. Talking more slowly also helps. Indeed, everything that slows down the pace of the confrontation has a calming effect. 'Wait a minute Mary. I am not understanding you well. Tell me what is happening.' A variation on this is to leave your patient alone for a while, and return, say, 15 minutes later in order to check whether or not his mood has changed.

Whatever tactic you choose, one thing is essential: you must stay calm.

Anger is never caused by an event or by something done by someone else: anger is caused solely by the thoughts an event provokes in our own minds. If you think 'He is doing that on purpose', you will feel anger. If, on the other hand, you think 'He can't help it, his illness is to blame', then it is unlikely that you will feel any annoyance at all. Breathing slowly and counting to ten will do the rest.

If nothing helps, sedatives can always be prescribed for the patient. They are, however, a last resort. (Unfortunately, many care institutions opt too readily for this solution to the problem.)

Aggression in someone with dementia is often viewed in a purely negative light. However understandable this might be, it is never entirely justified. Aggression can also be seen as having a positive side to it: it is a clear signal that the person concerned is unwilling to capitulate to his illness. It is an indication that he has not resigned himself to the fact that he makes mistakes. Aggression is his protest against his lot. Anyone still in possession of the small remains of his self-determination, or the last remnants of his self-esteem, will inevitably stubbornly resist his own on-going mental deterioration. It is more normal than abnormal that someone in the process of dementia will mobilize all the powers he still has to put up a strong and noble fight against what life has dealt him. And it is no wonder that he takes it out on everything and everyone around him. He cannot get a grip on his illness – all he can do is give vent to his profound displeasure and defiance where, and with whom, he is.

Here are a few more tips on how best to respond to aggression:

- Listen more than you speak.

- Allow your partner/relative with dementia to walk or move around (so that he can release some tension) before speaking to him.

- Ask him what it is he wants from you.

- Ensure that you are not blocking his path in any way (the feeling of being trapped can provoke and increase aggression).

Depressiveness

In Bernlef's novel *Out of mind* (1988), the main character's wife asks her husband Maarten one day how he is feeling. He replies:

> 'Like a ship, …a sailing ship with no wind in its sails. And then suddenly there is wind, and I set sail again. And then the world takes me in its grasp again, and I can move again with it.'
>
> 'It is so difficult to imagine, Maarten. I just can't see it in you. It's as if you are looking at something, something I can't see. Are you afraid at those moments? What is going on inside you exactly?'
>
> 'I don't know. I don't remember. Just that feeling of sudden blackness, as if I am sinking, and there is nothing I can hold on to.'
>
> (p.70)

How would you feel if you were experiencing what Maarten was experiencing?

People who have suffered a stroke which has affected the 'language centre' of the brain are often not able to find the words they need to express their thoughts. They might say, for instance, 'Could you give me a spoon, please?', whereas what they actually want is a fork. They hear themselves saying the wrong word – they see it coming, as it were – but can do nothing to stop it. Most people suffering from this disorder – aphasia – often have moments of deep melancholy. People with dementia often struggle with the same problem of finding the right word when they need it.

Ask yourself how you would feel if, as regularly happens to people with dementia, you have to search – in vain – for the right word. How would you feel if you regularly find yourself losing track of a thought, just when you are about to put it into words? It is rather like an angler seeing his catch slipping out of his fingers just as he is taking it off the hook.

Here we have another thought-experiment. You are in your shed, trying to repair the burst tyre on your bike, but you unexpectedly notice that all those familiar tools you have used all your life are suddenly not doing what you want them to do. Or you are in the kitchen, and you find yourself unable to do simple and familiar things in proper sequence. At a certain point you get 'stuck' and you don't know how to proceed.

How would you feel in this situation?

Helplessness and anxiety

Depressiveness, like aggression, is very often an expression of helplessness and anxiety. When someone constantly sees that he fails in practically everything he does, and he realizes at the same time that the cause of the failure lies in himself, then it will probably not leave him unmoved. Someone who, prior to the onset of the brain disorder, did not possess an abundance of self-esteem might well be tempted – as he always was – to vent his frustration on himself. He becomes angry with himself – and depression follows. In actual fact, depressiveness is always a reflection of anger turned in on itself. An aggressive person spits his fury out at those around him, whilst a depressive person shouts at himself: 'I'm no good, an idiot, a fool.'

These expressions of depressiveness will be most severe at moments when the person with dementia is most aware of his own condition. This will, as mentioned already in Chapter 1, be particularly apparent in the early phase of Alzheimer's. In the case of the less common multi-infarct dementia, however, it will persist well into the care-need period (the middle phase).

The core of every case of depressiveness lies in the huge gap that develops between desire and reality. Something is happening to the partner/relative with dementia and he does not like it – he does *not want* it. Or, by the same token, something he does want is *not happening.* He wants to go home, for instance, but he cannot remember how to do that. And he doesn't even know how he can make his wish clear to those around him.

Approach

One depressive person with dementia will realize his deteriorating situation better than another, and the degree to which he is aware of this determines how he should be approached. A strategy such as distraction will usually have a converse effect on those who know only too well the kind of mistakes they are making; for someone with a limited awareness of his disorder, however, distracting tactics can often produce the desired results. If you try to sidetrack someone who is aware of his mental deterioration, you leave him emotionally out in the cold. He feels he is not being taken seriously, and as a result of that his despair can become even greater. In all such cases, signs of true understanding and empathy are more appropriate and more effective. 'You look so unhappy. Are you okay?' Acknowledging and accepting personal emotions are primary and necessary steps towards helping someone at odds with himself. Being honest about our feelings can quite often clear the air for us. 'It makes me unhappy to see your suffering.' If he is unhappy because he has lost something, you could say something like: 'I hate not being able to help you find what is so important for you.'

In order to be able to console and stand by someone in his need, one does not always need to know the reason for his unhappiness. We can often do absolutely nothing about the cause of the depression, and asking about it will (again) embarrass and unsettle him, because he too is unable to give it a name. Finally, he may also feel a strong need to keep the explanation of his illness to himself. Precious moments can be lost in devoting frantic efforts to getting behind the cause of our partner's disquiet – and we can make far better use of those moments by simply 'being there' for him. Real concern and attention need not necessarily be expressed in words. People with dementia are often comforted by a gentle touch (an arm around his shoulders, for instance), by stroking his arm or back, by sitting next to him, by turning towards him, or by seeking direct eye contact. In this way, you indicate to him that you really do want to give him your help and support. It is extremely important for the dementia patient to know that there is someone on whom he can rely, and that he means something to that person too. The feeling of not being written off and the knowledge that the other really cares are the best antidotes to despondency.

Having managed to console your partner/relative with dementia, you can then attempt to turn his thoughts to other things. The depressive person – in the same way as someone who is depressive but does not have dementia – is not helped by being allowed to wallow in his gloominess.

There are several ways of distracting him from his sorrow. You can, for instance, turn his attention to a subject which you know will lighten his spirit, such as a favourite hobby or activity. Someone who used to enjoy skating, for instance, will probably perk up considerably by the very thought of gliding over the ice again; and a woman who regards her time as a domestic servant as the happiest period of her life will usually forget her tears when reminded of it.

> Mrs Klein is in the sitting room, sitting at a high table and crying uncontrollably. Nurse: 'Oh, Mrs Klein, come here. What is the matter? Come and sit on the couch with me for a while. Come and sit close to me.' The nurse walks to

the couch with the resident. The resident cuddles up to her. The nurse kisses her hair gently: 'Tell me what it is…' Sobbing Mrs Klein tells a story about Betty (her daughter) and her children. When she tells something about her husband the nurse asks: 'How long have you been married now?' Mrs Klein: 'For a long time.' Nurse: 'How old were you when you got married?' Mrs Klein: 'A bit older, 25 years at least.' 'Well, I was 32 years old,' the nurse says, 'even older than you were. And was he your first boyfriend?' Resident: 'No, I could get one for every day of the week. That was because I sang so beautifully.' Nurse: 'Sing something for us, Mrs Klein, please.' For a moment she hesitates, swallows another few tears and starts singing a ballad in a high voice. Everyone is listening quietly and attentively and spontaneously starts cheering when she stops singing. Mrs Klein is glowing.

(De Lange 2004)

Being active and busy also has a positive effect on someone's mood, although it has to be said immediately that it is often very difficult to stimulate a depressed person to undertake any kind of activity. The literal meaning of depression is 'downcast': people suffering from depression would *like* to be active but *cannot*. They feel as if they are glued to the ground under their feet, or that in order to do anything at all they have to wade through thick mud. Whilst the aggressive person has energy in abundance and is obsessed with the desire to have everything his own way, someone in a state of depression has to wrestle with his own incapacity to take on any task, however insignificant. It costs him enormous effort to come out of his cage.

If it is asking too much of your patient to take some real steps in this direction, you could suggest going to watch others busying themselves with some kind of activity or hobby.

'Would you like me to take you to the day room? No, you don't have to do anything. Just watch, okay?' This is sometimes sufficient, in itself, to win him over, and ultimately – via a detour – to get him actually to participate.

Giving compliments is also a well-proven method of boosting someone's morale: 'your hair looks lovely', or 'you look very smart today'.

Laughter, too, often has an amazing effect on someone's general mood. Laughter inspires laughter. Some people with dementia positively 'glow' with pleasure when greeted with a smile. Others come alive, as it were, if someone stops for a moment to talk with them – about the things around them, for instance, such as a bird busily looking for food on the lawn. The very fact that someone is talking to him gives the person with dementia the feeling that he really matters, even for a moment. And that is – as we commented earlier – often the best way of blowing away the dark clouds of unhappiness that seem constantly to envelop him.

Depression

This is a memory I have of my father's depression:

> During a certain period of his process of dementia my father was very down. While he had been very lively and energetic all of his life, he would now sit and stare gloomily for days and nothing would cheer him up. More than once he said, crying and screaming at my mother or my younger brothers and sisters still living at home, 'Get an axe out of the barn and chop my head off.'

When the sombreness is severe and persistent – longer than two weeks – and the person concerned is obviously burdened by it for most of every day, and all attempts to bring him out of it have little or no effect, it is probably no longer a question of depressiveness but rather of depression. This is a serious psychiatric disorder which is often accompanied by dementia. The cause can, in the same way as depressiveness, lie in the person's own awareness of the situation he is in. A heavy personal loss, the death of a partner for instance, can also provoke a depression. People who have had earlier periods of depression or some other psychiatric disorder run a higher risk of developing a combination of depression and dementia. The same is true for people with a first-degree relative (brother, sister, father, mother, child) who is suffering, or has suffered, from depression.

Depression provokes such a high degree of psychological suffering that people who have suffered from it tell us that there are no words that can truly describe the pain of it. Professional help should always be sought – for example, a general practitioner, a geriatrician or a psychiatrist – if there is any hint or suspicion of depression in your patient. There are medicines available now that can work very effectively in most cases of depression, and treatment can greatly improve both the patient's general mood and his overall ability to function.

Suspiciousness

Imagine that you feel that something is not quite right in you. You can't say exactly what it is, and you do not have a name for it. There are moments when you feel totally swamped by a kind of despair you have never felt before. At other moments, you feel completely alone, as if everyone has abandoned you. You feel extremely forlorn. You need your partner now more than ever before. Without her you cannot cope. Sometimes suddenly, and out of nowhere, you find yourself throttled by the fearful thought that she is going to leave you. What have you got to offer her, anyway? Your former strength seems to have seeped out of your body. You are dependent on her in so many ways. You might say it openly, but you really do feel terribly dependent on her. And there is something else: she leaves the house more frequently, and without saying anything to you (or you cannot remember her saying anything).

Where is she going? Has she found someone else? One day you look outside and you see your wife talking to your neighbour – he and she are talking and laughing together. You are afraid and jealous, and you say to yourself: 'I don't have to take this.' You rush outside and call your wife to order: 'You vulgar woman, you slut.' You know that what you are saying is not acceptable, but your fury is so great that you cannot control it. Your anger is as great as your fear of losing her. In the ensuing days, the only thought churning through your mind is: 'My wife is going to leave me.' (The vehemence of the emotion ensures that the thought – despite serious memory problems – is well and truly locked in your head.)

You fire accusations at her at the slightest provocation. 'Go and see your boyfriend next door,' you say. And your greatest fear is that she will do just that. You denounce her for no other reason than you want to be reassured and hear her say: 'But, John dear, don't worry yourself. You are the only man I love. I need you.'

Suppose you are in an area which is not familiar to you. The building you are in is like no other building you have ever seen before. The people around you are also strange. You do not know any of them; and they are all the same age! If they say something, you very often do not understand what they are talking about. You ask yourself: 'How did I come to be here?' One thing is absolutely certain: you do not belong here. You want to leave; but no matter how long you search for it, you cannot find the exit. If you do find a door, it's locked. What's behind it? Something is not right.

Or imagine you have always been someone oozing self-confidence. If you were successful at something, you attributed it entirely to your own efforts and abilities. If something did not go well, however, you could hardly conceive that you might have had a role in it. Your attitude prompted some people, therefore, to see you as conceited and arrogant. And then you become forgetful, but you are scarcely aware of it. That there is something amiss with your mind does not fit the image you have of yourself. And yet you regularly notice that things are not going as you would wish. You feel for your wallet in your inside pocket, but it's not there. But it was always there! As ever, you do not doubt yourself for one moment. It doesn't enter your head for a second that you might have put your wallet somewhere else. You think 'It wasn't me, so it must have been someone else', and because there is only one other person in the house – your partner – she must be the one to blame.

Backgrounds

More than half of our dementia sufferers have exhibited suspicion symptoms for longer or shorter periods of time. They lack confidence in others to an exceptionally high degree.

Memory loss as a result of dementia leads inevitably – as we pointed out earlier – to all kinds of failures and mistakes. These, in turn, provoke feelings of uncertainty, anxiety and panic. Apart from aggression and depressiveness, the person with dementia can respond to these feelings with deep suspicion. Suspicion is actually the cunning brother of aggression. The message the aggressive person with dementia is sending out is 'I am very angry that this is happening to me', whilst the suspicious person adds yet another subtle layer to the complaint, in terms of: 'I am not the cause of this awful situation – you are.'

People who tended in the past to be dominant and excessively self-confident are more likely to react in this way. It has, after all, always been their way of dealing with uncertainties and setbacks. They were somewhat mistrustful by nature in the past too, and they have now simply 'upped' the level of that doubt by several degrees.

There are also many people who were previously neither exceptionally self-assured nor distrustful, but who have now developed a suspicious trait, as a result of their inability to judge or command the situation in which they now find themselves. Lack of knowledge combined with anxiety, uncertainty and feelings of insecurity constitute the ideal breeding ground for fantasies and imagined 'schemes', the main thrust being: 'Others are up to no good, but they don't fool me.' An example of this is a woman with dementia who catches a fragment of a conversation her husband is having with their eldest daughter. She clearly hears the words 'old people's home', and the fear grabs her by the throat that her husband and her daughter want to put her into a home. That's why they have been nagging at her so often lately!

Approach

The first thing that needs to be done when someone with dementia utters some kind of accusation is to check whether or not it is true. The fact that someone is suffering from dementia does not mean that we should automatically disbelieve him. A person with dementia who says he is being mistreated or that, for example, his wallet has been stolen from him is not always lying. If you are the target of his mistrust, it is of course easy enough to know whether or not he is speaking the truth. If his accusation is unfounded, however, it is wise to inform those around him so that they will be prepared for something similar. This will also make things considerably easier for the patient's relatives, friends, carers or home-help, as well as himself. How should we respond to the person pointing the finger of suspicion – that is, the person with dementia? Just as in the case of aggression, it is better not to respond to the content of the accusation, but rather to the message behind it: his feelings. Suppose someone says: 'You have stolen my razor.' An obvious reaction would be to deny the accusation, but all you are doing in this case is adding fuel to the fire. It would be better to say: 'I can see that you are very upset. Everything and everyone seems to be against you. Let's start looking for your razor now.' With this type of response, you short-change neither yourself (you admit no guilt) nor your partner/relative with dementia (you are not lying to him).

This kind of approach will not usually help, however, in the case of the person with dementia accusing you of being someone else. The worst kinds of profanities are being thrown at you, and you discover that your patient sees you as the cousin with whom he had a terrible clash some 40 years ago. Hearing your voice will sometimes help in this situation, but often there is nothing else to do but allow your patient to blast off steam – just let it happen. Trying to enter into a discussion about it will only make things worse. Another possibility is to leave your patient alone for a while, in the hope that the thunder clouds will pass.

To be wrongfully accused is very painful indeed, and certainly when the accusations are so completely off the mark. It is important, however, not to blame your partner/relative himself, but rather his illness. In this case, accusations are not directed primarily to the person in sight; they are more the voice of protest against the situation in which he unwillingly finds himself. 'You are unkind to me' actually means 'Life is unkind to me'.

Here are a few more tips on how to deal with suspicion:

- Avoid accentuating your patient's mistakes and mishaps, and do everything possible to present the message that everything is okay or that everything will be alright.

- Check whether your patient is seeing and hearing well. Deafness and poor vision can easily lead to wrong interpretations and to the feeling of being left out.

- Avoid whispering.

- Check whether or not the patient's medication is causing the suspicious attitude. Anti-Parkinson medication, for instance, is known to provoke suspicious thinking from time to time. Inform your patient's doctor.

- Inform anyone who comes into contact with the partner/relative with dementia about his tendency to be suspicious. This will prevent them believing the accusations made against you, or from abandoning him if, and when, they too become the target of his abuse.

- Try to draw your patient's thoughts away from what is troubling him by, for example, singing one of his favourite songs.

6

Behaviour problems
Clinging behaviour, wandering and nocturnal restlessness

Introduction

In this chapter, we will discuss behaviour problems which can often go hand in hand with dementia. We will focus on three problems in particular which often cause the most stress for relatives and carers: clinging behaviour, wandering and nocturnal restlessness.

For the family members, it is important once again to bear in mind that behaviour of this kind can be symptomatic of the illness itself. The person directly concerned cannot help what he is doing and there is no point, therefore, in repeatedly drawing his attention to it.

Clinging behaviour: 'He follows me around like a shadow'

John Bayley wrote the following about his wife, Iris Murdoch:

> A goose which cannot find other geese will attach itself to some object – another animal, even a stone or a post – and

never lose sight of it. This terror of being alone, of being cut off for even a few seconds from the familiar object, is a feature of Alzheimer's. If Iris could climb inside my skin now, or enter me as if I had a pouch like a kangaroo, she would do so.

(Bayley 1999)

Astronauts who have been a crew member of a long-haul space flight often say on their return to earth that it was not homesickness, weightlessness or the lack of amusement that was the most difficult aspect of the whole venture, but rather the fact that they were never alone, even for a few moments. Privacy is one of the most elementary human needs. Nearly every adult needs a moment when he can do whatever he wants, without feeling someone else's eyes on him. The dementia patient, however, will often not leave his caring partner/relative alone for one second and he will not want to be left alone either. Before going more deeply into this so-called clinging behaviour, I would like to invite our readers to take part in the following thought-experiment.

Suppose you are walking in an area with which you are unfamiliar. Let's say in a fairly remote region of Scotland. You follow the hikers' route which is indicated by splashes of paint on trees, stones, lantern poles and bridges. After walking for three hours, you suddenly realize you have lost your way. To make matters worse, a thick mist is descending all around you. It is so misty, in fact, that you can hardly see more than five metres ahead. Fortunately, however, you are not alone. You have a companion who has a torch, a detailed map and a compass. Your companion doesn't panic for a second. It is absolutely clear that he is in total control of the situation. Despite the mist and despite having wandered away from the track, you feel quite safe. And then – all of a sudden – your travelling companion has disappeared. You call his name, but there is no answer. You feel your heart thumping. You start to sweat. And because you don't know what to do, you start walking round in ever-decreasing circles. You lose all sense of time. You have only one thing on your mind: where has my travelling companion gone? And then he reappears just as suddenly as he disappeared. He is back.

What a relief! You are actually so relieved that you forget to be angry. Yet that feeling of panic and desperation continues to echo for a long time in your head.

Ask yourself how you would continue this journey. More specifically: how careful would you be about keeping a close eye on your travelling companion from then on?

Deep-seated feelings of uncertainty/insecurity

The clinging behaviour so common among dementia patients arises from a fundamental sense of uncertainty or insecurity and is caused by a memory box disintegrating on all sides. People in the early stages of dementia simply do not know their way around in their own lives any more and are very often largely unable to understand what is going on around them. Intuitively, however, they are aware that the person caring for them is the one who *does* know what is going on, and if that person is absent for some reason, dementia patients will immediately feel very uneasy indeed.

The disorientation in time means that someone with dementia is hardly able to judge how much time has passed – he also experiences time differently from us. One minute can seem like an hour to him. Just as a toddler feels perfectly safe so long as he can see his mother (or father), the dementia patient only feels comfortable and safe so long as his carer remains within his field of vision. 'Better safe than sorry' is his motto.

Interaction

The kind of feelings a carer might experience when being constantly followed around by someone in a state of dementia might include: 'What he is really hoping for is attention', 'He doesn't want to keep himself occupied', or 'He doesn't trust me, and that's why he keeps an eye on me all the time.' There is a big difference, however, between this kind of thinking, and knowing the true reasons that lie behind this very annoying kind of behaviour: the reasons are anxiety and uncertainty, which in turn are the consequences of a failing memory.

To avoid clinging behaviour, the carer will need – at as early a stage as possible – to ensure that the patient becomes accustomed to the fact that several people will be involved in his care. Thus – in the phase within which he is still able to learn – he should be told that the carer/relative performing the central (caring) role will not always be with him. The aim here is to help him feel equally secure with others.

If this advice cannot be put into practice then there is still a good alternative: the idea is to prevent or diminish the dementia patient's fear of being left in the lurch. The carer should say in advance why he/she is going to leave the room; for instance: 'I'm just going upstairs to make the beds', or 'I'm just going to do a quick chore in the garden.' In some cases it helps if – before moving from the patient's room to another, or before leaving the house to do some shopping, for instance – a video is set to run on which the patient can see and hear the carer. In that case, the carer is still 'at least partially present' for him. (The carer should also ensure that a reserve door key is always available, or that it is hidden in a safe place outside the house. This will prevent the added hassle of being locked out!) As long as the dementia patient can still read or tell the time, it is always possible for you, as a carer, to write on a piece of paper or a blackboard near him – before leaving him – where you are going and when you will be back.

For your own peace of mind, it might also be possible sometimes to stimulate the patient to occupy himself with worthwhile activities or hobbies. If you regularly take an interest in what he is doing, or help him deal with any problems that arise, or praise him for his efforts, you will be less bothered by the feeling of his 'constantly breathing down your neck'.

There is often no one solution which can be relied upon to work effectively in all circumstances, as far as dementia behaviour problems are concerned. It is usually a question of just being realistic and making do. Sometimes the only thing to be done is to share the discomfort and the disquiet. There is no escaping the fact that a dementia patient will have to be left alone at various times of the day, and there is no escaping the fact that he will not want it – the carer, too, has to surrender more privacy and freedom than he or she would like. There is, after all, no medicine for every pain.

Wandering

> I had just gone upstairs to make the bed, and when I came down again my husband was nowhere to be seen. I had forgotten to lock the back door, and he had obviously made his escape through it. When I went outside and called his name, there was no response. I immediately jumped onto my bike and went in search of him. In vain. I was getting more and more worried and anxious. Six hours later, I received a telephone call from a woman I did not know who told me that my husband was sitting in her pub. It appeared that he had covered a distance of some 15 kilometres. Via a narrow lane which runs alongside the

railway line, he had reached the area in which he was born and brought up. There he found his childhood home, a farmhouse which the present owners had turned into a pub some 30 years before, and he walked in. A former neighbour and acquaintance had recognized him.

(A wife)

The tendency for dementia patients to walk out of the door and wander around endlessly is a very difficult problem, for those close to them, to control. This kind of physical activity on the patient's part causes worry and fear in the minds of those responsible for his care and well-being, and sometimes considerable irritation as well; worry and fear, in terms of the risks of his falling, or of accidents, or even of his becoming totally exhausted; irritation is also possible because the carers themselves can become restless in the face of the patient's restlessness, or because of the continuous pressure his behaviour puts on everything and everyone around him.

Causes

Wandering as dementia patients tend to do is actually just like every other kind of behaviour, in the sense that it too has a meaning and a purpose, and can usually be related back to one or more of the following causes. Some dementia patients are unable to sit still for long because they are simply 'brimming over with energy'. Although dementia often makes patients more apathetic and passive than they had been before the illness started, in others the very opposite is true and their self-control disappears and they cannot quieten the irresistible urge to go for a walk. This enormous and pressing need to do a walkabout is especially evident in dementia patients who are otherwise healthy and physically fit.

It might be that walking helps the patient to deal, in part at least, with his anxieties and all the other emotions which bother him so much; that is, physical exercise is a means of releasing physical and emotional tension. The same is also true for 'normal' healthy people in times of stress.

In some cases, the dementia patient's need to walk is nothing more than a reflection of the fact that during his working life he was on his feet for most of the day: he might have been a waiter, a farmer, a barber, a postman, or a football trainer. His need to walk now, therefore, is simply an extension of his former way of life.

Wanting to take a walk could also relate to physical restlessness caused by pain, obstipation or medication (such as tranquillizers having a counter-productive effect). Some patients become over-active as a result of medication not working as it should, and sometimes to an almost maniacal extent. They cannot sit still for a single moment and are hardly able even to settle down long enough to take a meal. The urge to walk can also be provoked by pleasing stimulants, such as coffee, cigarettes, social contacts, or a lovely view.

On the other hand, the continual urge to roam and wander might also arise from the dementia patient's need to escape from the environment around him which he perceives as unpleasant and undesirable. Some such people never, or hardly ever, join their fellow residents in the main sitting-room of the care home they share, because – as they themselves put it – they 'do not want to sit with all those loonies'!

Before we move on to the last cause of wandering behaviour, it might help if we did another thought-experiment.

Imagine that at the age of 75 you step into a time-machine which takes you 65 years back in time. Suddenly you are ten years old again. The time-machine, however, has *not* turned back the time for the environment you knew so well all those years ago. You look around and recognize nothing. You ask yourself: 'Where is my mother, where is our house?'

Now ask yourself this: do you stay where you are, or do you explore?

The last – frequently occurring – cause of wandering behaviour is, thus, the dementia patient's perception that the environment in which he finds himself is unfamiliar to him. He is living in the past, sometimes as far back as 60 or 70 years ago. His wandering urges, therefore, have a definite purpose: he wants to be somewhere else. He is searching for his birthplace, his family home, his parents. He is, literally and figuratively speaking, definitely not 'at home' in his present environment.

Approach

In order to deal with his wandering, the carer needs to find an approach that connects with the cause of the patient's need to wander off. The first question you need to ask, however, is: is the wandering habit bothersome or dangerous? If it is purely bothersome – the early-stage dementia patient is, after all, still able to find his way home again – then there is no real problem at all. If the situation is indeed problematical, however, then you – the main carer – will need to do everything possible to discover the cause. Each type of wandering or walking-around behaviour demands a different approach.

If the monotonous pacing back and forth, roaming through the rooms of the house, or rattling the door handle are an expression of the patient's need to have his daily portion of exercise, then the solution is obvious: take a walk with him once or twice a day, and allow him to busy himself with something else which will help to occupy his mind and dissipate his energy. A home-trainer can sometimes help in this situation. Access to a daycare centre for dementia patients can often bring welcome respite, especially when the caregiver is carrying sole responsibility for the patient's care and well-being. In most nursing homes, walking-around-for-the-sake-of-walking-around is usually not a problem. New nursing homes, especially, incorporate this need into their building plans, thereby enabling their residents to walk around endlessly, and to their heart's content.

If, as carer, you suspect that the cause of the physical restlessness lies in some kind of physical disorder – obstipation, for instance – then you will need to discuss it with your patient's doctor.

If the search for effective stimuli, or the avoidance of undesired stimuli, proves to be the motor behind the dementia patient's behaviour, there are still ways in which you can help him. The key might lie in structured activities, for instance, linked directly to his own interests, and carried out in a pleasing and relaxed atmosphere.

It is much more difficult to find the best approach if the walking and wandering is an expression of the patient's determined efforts to be somewhere else. Experimentation is often the answer here. The first option is to allow your patient to do what he wants to do and, for safety reasons, to go with him. Once you are outside and have walked, cycled or driven for a while, the patient himself will very often indicate that he wants to go back to where he came from. We realize, of course, that this solution is not always workable in either the home or nursing home situation. Relatives usually do not have the time or the energy to take on the extra task of going for long walks with their patient once or twice a day, on top of all the other daily care requirements.

Another way of getting a grip on this type of wandering behaviour is to apply the strategy of combining empathetic listening with distraction tactics. The first step is gain eye contact with your patient, and then take him gently by the arm (if he will allow it), and ask him what he wants. The point here is to get behind what is driving him. You then pick out the most important words or phrases contained in his reply: 'milk the cows', 'the children are home from school', 'cook the meal'. It is even better to try to put the dementia patient's feelings into words: 'you are missing your mother', or 'you are worried that the cows are not going to be milked today'. Whilst you are talking in this way, you gently lead him, almost imperceptibly, in the desired (other) direction. If this does not work, you can try to dampen his desire to go for a walk by continuing the strategy of repeating words and phrases in the search for his underlying feelings. A little later you can then try to bring him back on track: 'let's walk this way'. And you can often combine this method with 'white lies': 'Mum and Dad are not home today because they have gone to see Uncle John', or 'There's no need to worry, your sons Dick and Rod have already milked the cows.' Of course it is also possible to combine the strategies mentioned (both make the patient move and distract him).

> He always wanted to go away. He could enjoy himself, but at a certain moment he would stand up and say: 'Now I am going home.' 'Home' was his own home, to his mother, to his father. It took a lot of creativity to handle this. What was best was to literally walk along with him until he was really tired and started going back. Or we said: 'The car broke down', or 'That is not possible now, the train has just left.' That worked, he would come back then. It was absolutely no use to use the weather as an argument by saying it was too cold or too hot. You had to go outside with him and walk with him until he was tired. At the end he became tired very quickly, after about 300 metres. 'I will go tomorrow,' he would say then.
>
> (Avontroodt 2002)

If nothing at all helps and you are afraid the person with dementia will wear himself out with all his walking and wandering, then there are various medications available which will subdue and relax him, in the hope that his wandering urges will also decrease. The danger here, however, is that these medicines carry an increased risk of accidents or falls; that is, they can affect a person's concentration, stability and/or balance. In this case – as is so often the case in caring for someone in the process of dementia – we have to opt for whichever is the lesser of two evils.

Emergency measures

It is impossible, in the home situation, for a carer to keep a permanent eye on the comings and goings of the person with dementia in his/her care. If you want to protect him from his wanderings, and spare yourself the task of searching for him, then there is no alternative but to lock all doors. If you want to be absolutely certain that he will not 'escape', then you can fix new locks with which he is unfamiliar. The risk that the dementing patient will find his way out of the house is thus very small indeed bearing in mind that his failing memory will prevent him from understanding how the new locks work. Another suggestion is to place the locks higher or lower on the door – your patient will be less inclined to look for them there. Some people with dementia can be kept safely in the house by hiding the things they always reach for when going for a walk. For one this might be a hat, for another a walking stick, and for someone else the favourite walking shoes. These are obviously not very 'elegant' measures, but they are sometimes very necessary. An alarm system could also be installed if you feel a real need to prevent your patient from slipping out of the house unseen. There are alarm systems, for instance, which are placed under the mat by the back and front doors and are activated as soon as someone treads on them. If that is too expensive, a simple clanging bell can be fixed to the back and front doors which rings loud and clear whenever the door is opened. Window locks are also recommended, and any automatic doors (garage doors, for instance) should be put entirely out of use.

It is also advisable to ensure that your patient does not carry large sums of money on his person, so that if – despite all the preventive measures that have been put in place – he still manages to 'escape', there will be no serious financial damage. Ensure too that he always carries a card bearing his name, address and telephone number – in his purse or on an SOS-medallion attached to a chain around his neck, or to a watch or bracelet (the latter engraved with name, address and telephone number is another possibility). Identification information can also be embroidered (or written) on a piece of cloth which is then sewn into the inside of a coat or jacket, and, in order to make your patient more 'visible' on the street, reflection tape can also be attached to his outdoor clothing.

In villages, most people know each other, and most of them will know, therefore, who among them is suffering from dementia. Because this is far less likely to happen in a town or city, however, it is worth informing local people about your patient's mental condition. These people might include shop-keepers, publicans or the local 'bobby', and providing them with a recent photograph (or video clip, if possible) of the person concerned can also be very useful.

Nocturnal restlessness

If your wife gets up at half past two in the morning, and then puts on three layers of clothing over her nightdress (and allows her own urine to drench it all), you might

think you can save the situation by talking to her *v-e-r-y
s-l-o-w-l-y* and *v-e-r-y c-l-e-a-r-l-y*. You take her by the arm
and lead her to the window in the lounge and you say:
'My dear girl, my darling Susan – take a look outside. The
street lamps are still on, there is no one to be seen, there
are no lights in the houses, everyone is asleep. So come on
my love, let's go to sleep too.' And then she looks at you as
if she wants to say: 'You're mad – what kind of crazy
world are YOU living in?!'

(Vergoed 1993)

Sleeping problems, and the nocturnal 'haunting' that ensues
from them, occur very often in cases of dementia. A possible
cause of this – for the family – very tiring form of behaviour
has to do with the first law of dementia, namely the inability to
absorb impressions or information. As it is not easy to see
the connection between this and nocturnal wanderings, the
following thought-experiment has been devised to illustrate
the link.

Disturbed information absorption

Imagine that – just like someone with dementia – you are able
to remember things for just 30 seconds, and not a second
longer. This disaster has suddenly overcome you within the
space of a single day – let's say as a result of severe concussion
following a car accident. You go to bed at the normal time with
this very reduced memory span. You wake up at 4 a.m. Your
bladder is full, and you automatically reach for the light switch
above your bed and you stumble, more asleep than awake,
down the stairs on your way to the toilet – and when you have
finished you close the toilet door behind you. Thirty seconds
have passed in the meantime, and you are no longer aware of

the fact that less than a minute ago you were fast asleep in bed. You then notice that you are wearing your pyjamas and you draw the obvious conclusion: I am up, so I must have had my full night's sleep. You are thirsty and you decide to make yourself a cup of tea. And because the house is so quiet, you turn on the radio – you turn up the volume because there is no one else around anyway. Three minutes later, the telephone rings. It's the neighbour: 'Hey, what's going on – turning on the radio so loud at this hour?! Could you soften it a bit please? And, anyway, why aren't you in bed?'

Other causes

Apart from the breakdown of the information absorption process mentioned above, there are other possible explanations for nocturnal restlessness. It might be that painful emotions and thoughts rise to the surface at night and break the dementia patient's sleep. For people without dementia, most emotions are more intense during the evening and night-time hours than they are during the day, and it is not difficult to imagine, therefore, that this is equally true for dementia patients. Small daytime worries can turn into very big, sleep-disturbing, anxieties as darkness falls – for both people with dementia and people without dementia. When our sleep is disturbed we, like someone with dementia, climb out of bed and start to pace up and down in an effort to rid our bodies of all that tension and inexplicable restlessness.

Another explanation for nocturnal restlessness might be that for people suffering from dementia the distinction between waking, sleeping and dreaming is more diffuse. Perhaps, because of numbed physical sensitivity, they are less able to feel the difference between being tired and having had sufficient sleep.

It is also possible that a person with dementia becomes restless at night because he actually went to bed too early. Because the partner or resident carer would otherwise not have a moment to themselves all day, it could be that he/she has taken the step of 'tucking up the patient in bed' at too early an hour. (In care homes and nursing homes, residents are often in bed at 8 p.m., simply because there is insufficient personnel available to lift them into bed later in the evening.)

It might also be that the cause of nocturnal restlessness is primarily physiological by nature. For instance, the Dutch brain expert Professor Swaab discovered in the early 1990s that the biological clock in the brain – a tiny in-built human alarm clock – breaks down very early on in the dementia process.

A final explanation is that nocturnal restlessness may be a consequence of an excess or lack of certain chemical substances in the brain. It is known, for instance, that one neuro-transmitter (Noradrenaline) can cause depression as well as a tremendous need for sleep. There is often a significant shortage of this same neuro-transmitter in cases of Alzheimer's disease too, and this probably also explains why many dementia patients have no choice but to doze their way through the greater part of every day. Having 'nodded off' throughout the day it is no wonder that they tend to wake up from time to time during the night.

Approach

Nocturnal restlessness belongs to the problem category for which there is, unfortunately, no easy solution. In many situations it is impossible, it seems, to find any workable solution at all.

If nocturnal restlessness does occur, however, the most important thing to remember is to remain very calm. We realize, of course, that this is far easier said than done and that it affects relatives and partners alike. No one can be expected to be in the best of moods when robbed of sleep, and it means – just as in the case of the partner referred to at the beginning of this section – that it is even more difficult for a carer to muster the necessary self-control to deal with the situation. Keeping calm remains, nonetheless, the best course of action. Angry words and angry outbursts usually result in putting the dementia patient into a bad mood too – you then become even more 'heated' and any chance of getting back to sleep evaporates. What usually helps is to speak gently and calmly to the patient and then patiently lead him back to bed.

Nocturnal restlessness is best prevented, of course. The following measures, which are equally valid for people without dementia with sleeping problems, can often help dementia patients to have a good night's sleep:

- Avoid caffeine after 5 p.m.

- Consult the treating doctor and ask if medication might be the cause of the sleeplessness.

- Hang thick curtains in the bedroom; this helps prevent the dementia patient seeing the full moon, or the early light of dawn, as a sign that daytime has come and that it's time to get up.

- Ensure that he has a comfortable mattress, a good room temperature (not too hot and not too cold), and a good degree of air humidity.

- Ensure that his pyjamas are not too tight.

- Prevent the patient from turning day into night by not allowing him to doze off too often throughout the day.

- Take care that he does not have to absorb too many impressions or events that cost him extra mental and physical effort at the end of the day.

- Do everything possible to build up a set sleeping pattern by ensuring that your patient goes to bed at a certain time every day and is woken up at a set time every morning.

- We know, of course, that a glass of warm milk or alcohol can help all of us to drift gently into sleep. Too much alcohol, however – that is, more than two units, and for some people more than one unit – has a converse effect. It can cause early wake-ups and restless sleep for the person with dementia (as well as for the person without).

- Try to encourage the dementia patient to go to the toilet before going to bed. Place a night light next to his bed; this provides a reassuring orientation point and will prevent extra confusion and anxiety if he needs to go to the toilet during the night. It is worth noting, however, that many older people have no problem at all in using a chamber pot, a commode or a urinal at their bedside.

- Ensure that his daytime clothing is out of sight and out of reach at night. Talking someone out of his clothes in the middle of the night can be a very exhausting undertaking. The best thing to do is lock the wardrobe.

- Sleeping tablets constitute the last remedy at our disposal. They must, however, only be used sporadically and never for longer than two or three weeks at a stretch. After that, they have the opposite effect and are also addictive.

(Buijssen and Razenberg 1991)

Radical measures

Sometimes nothing you attempt has any effect at all; however, if the recharging of our batteries is cruelly interrupted day after day, then even the most iron-willed of us will ultimately reach the point of total exhaustion. If the measures listed above do not help, then you will have to resort to more radical means. First, you should have your own bedroom (assuming you have not done this already) and, with earplugs firmly planted in your ears, you simply leave the dementia patient to do whatever he wants. A number of precautionary steps have to be taken in advance of this, however, so that the risk of accidents can be kept to a minimum.

A second possibility is that you try to get some daytime sleep too: when your partner, for instance, is at the day centre, or when he himself is having his customary afternoon 'nap'.

A third possibility is to ask a relative, a good friend or someone from a voluntary organization to act as night-watch from time to time. During that time you will sleep at another address – in the house of the relative who is standing in for you that night, for instance.

A final possibility is to use the services of a (temporary) night-nurse. Some nursing homes offer this facility, precisely so that caregivers who are getting to the end of their tether as a result of the nocturnal restlessness can gather strength again and take stock.

7

Management guidelines and activities

Introduction

In the previous six chapters, we have tried to present useful advice on various aspects of interacting with people with dementia. In this chapter, we will put them into a working sequence, adding a few extra ideas at the same time. We will then present some guidelines on how best to embark on a programme of activities for/with your dementia patient, and we will close the chapter with a list of possible ways of keeping him pleasantly occupied.

Management guidelines

Memory boosters

In the case of early-stage dementia patients, it is worth trying to introduce them to activities which boost their memory capacities. You could, for instance, write a list of daily tasks in a notebook and ask your patient to draw a line through each task as he completes it. Important appointments should be written on a calendar.

If he is still living alone and is assisted by several carers, you can indicate in his notebook who will come and when; he will then know in advance who to expect and at what time. Telephone numbers which he needs to use regularly should be written on a piece of paper next to the telephone. A drawing, or photograph, of the bathroom and toilet can be pasted on the appropriate doors and will help your patient to find his way around.

Adapt to his pace

It is important to keep pace with your patient – everything works much more slowly for him now, so too his thinking process. It is worth remembering that dementia patients (almost) always immediately forget what they have seen and heard, and thus perceive most things as new and unfamiliar, whilst for us they are very familiar indeed. When a dementia patient dresses himself in the morning, his items of clothing are the first things he will want to inspect. They are not only things he is, apparently, seeing for the first time, but he first of all has to recognize them for what they are. He then has to discover which item of clothing it is: is it his trousers or is it his vest? And that's not the end of it. He still has to discover which trouser leg has to go on which leg – the right or the left? Whilst going through the procedure of getting dressed, it is not unusual for his disorientation in time to throw him completely off track. Does he have to get dressed now, or was he in the process of getting *un*dressed? And lastly, he is easily distracted because he tends to lose himself in tiny details. A female dementia patient, for instance, can become totally absorbed by the flower pattern on her blouse.

Take images and anxieties seriously

When you find a dementia patient hallucinating, the best thing you can do is calm him down by taking his images and anxieties seriously. Do not pretend that you can see and hear what he sees and hears, but try instead to reassure him by saying something like: 'I cannot see that strange man you see in the corner of the room, but I *can* see that he is frightening you.' The anxiety often disappears – at least temporarily – if you show you are prepared to take specific action to chase the images away, such as: 'Shall I go to the corner of the room and send the man away for you?'

In some cases the person with dementia can be encouraged to do something:

> She sometimes says: 'Last night a strange man slept next to me. You were not here. You went into town again.' I asked her: 'Who slept next to you then?' 'Well, an old man, I do not know who he was,' she said. Then I say: 'You should not let him, next time you should throw him out of bed, because he does not belong here.' I just make a joke of it. That is what I do.
>
> (A husband, quoted in Duijnstee 1996)

Inability to learn new things

Do not attempt to teach anything new to your dementia patient. This is a complete waste of energy. Activities which, until recently, he could undertake quite easily, but which have now become too complicated for him – making his bed, or eating with a knife and fork, for instance – cannot be re-learned now, for the simple reason that his memory span is far too short; his ability to recall fades rapidly. There is no point any more in trying to change someone's character. You will never succeed. Try, instead, to work with his character as it is, play on it. For proud individuals, for instance, well-chosen words can often work miracles. Instead of saying 'It's time for tea', try saying 'I have made us a nice cup of tea'. A sentence which begins with 'Would you like...?' often falls on more fruitful ground than a direct statement.

Avoid confrontation

Do not directly confront the person with dementia with his mistakes – this only causes upset and anger. This does not mean, however, that you have to ignore all his mistakes: you can correct him, but not in terms of: 'I keep telling you...' or 'How could you...?' If you want to put something right, do it in a calm and gentle manner, preferably as discreetly as possible so that he will not lose face.

Avoiding confrontation is an important issue in handling a family member with dementia, as is evident in the account of this husband who describes various ways in which he succeeds in preventing a situation from developing into a confrontation:

> Sometimes she says: 'What kind of funny food is this that we have got here?' and I just leave her be, I am not going to start nagging her to think about it. I just let her babble, that is the best you can do. If you contradict her, it only gets worse, the only time I sometimes argue with her is when she no longer recognizes me, then I say: 'I am B', but then again, sometimes I do not. Then she says: 'No, you are not my husband,' or something like that. That is my second life. Then I have to get her going from scratch again. I show her pictures and that sort of thing, and slowly it all comes back to her and she says: 'Oh yes, that is right.' Of course I always let her win when we are playing games and stuff, smart as I am. She then says: 'I won again, didn't I?' That is how I do that, and I also just go along with what she is saying. Across the street lives a man who is 60 years old and also has dementia. And every morning he and his wife take a stroll here and my wife

says: 'There is that man, he is as demented as can be, he is
crazy.' And I say: 'I am so glad you are still well.'

(Quoted in Duijnstee 1996)

Order, regularity and rest

Patients with dementia have a great need for order, regularity
and rest. Try to satisfy this need as much as possible and
establish a set daily routine, such as: get up, get washed and
dressed, have breakfast, do some shopping, have a cup of
coffee, take a rest, do small jobs in the house, have lunch, go for
a walk, tidy up, take a snooze, have a cup of tea, prepare the
meal, have an aperitif, have your evening meal, relax, go to
sleep.

Bearing in mind that dementia is usually accompanied by
disorientation in terms of place, you should be very careful
when introducing changes into his immediate environment.
Ensure that the furniture remains where it has always been.
Keep things uncluttered in the house so that your patient can
take it all in at one glance, and ensure that he can easily locate
the things that are important to him.

Try to avoid unfamiliar situations and a programme that is
too busy for him – it can unsettle him and make him uneasy. Do
not press him if you notice something is causing him too much
tension – he will only become even more confused. Remember
that responses to stressful situations will not always be
immediate; they may, in fact, only be manifested some time
later, in such ways as difficulty in falling asleep, nocturnal
restlessness, or extra confusion or tiredness the following day.

Do not demand too much nor too little

Continue to address those things of which the person with
dementia is still capable. This is essential if his self-respect is to

be sustained. It is not a good idea to take something out of his hands just because he does it too slowly, or because he cannot do it 100 per cent successfully. All of us, the dementia patient too, needs to feel capable – indeed, it is the basis on which our self-esteem is largely built. Maybe the person with dementia can't dress himself as routinely as he used to, but he is well able nonetheless to put on some items of clothing without help. He can be helped considerably and his memory jogged, for instance, by having his clothes laid out in the right order in advance, and by calmly being given the necessary instructions. Help him when he needs it. This latter point is important because over-questioning is just as bad as under-questioning. What matters is getting the right balance.

To determine what you can ask from someone with dementia, it is advisable to take someone's past into account:

> Andrea was a 27-year-old nurse. Soon she would get married. She was the nurse responsible for a man in his early seventies. He had mild dementia and suffered heavily from pulmonary emphysema. He was not willing to do much for himself and expected the nurses to do everything for him. Therefore there was a constant negative atmosphere between the nurses and this man. The nurses thought he could do more for himself if he wanted to. Andrea kind of liked him and thought about it. She came to the conclusion that the man reminded her of her grandfather, who had been pampered by her grandmother all his life. And actually her mother had done the same thing: her father just had to say something and her mother would come running to him helpfully. She herself could not be absolved either: she was constantly cleaning up after her boyfriend. Once she had realized this, she decided to just take care of the man as his wife had used to, but to try and change things in her own

life. The result was that the man became very fond of her and did more for her than for the nurses who tried to impose their will on him.

(Van der Kooy 2003)

Treat him as an adult

Take the person with dementia seriously and *treat him as an adult*. A person bothered by loss of decorum can also feel embarrassed – when undressing before taking a shower, for instance. He also knows only too well when you are talking about him with someone else in his presence. Allow him to keep his wallet; being in possession of money adds to his sense of being secure. It need not be a large sum, of course. For someone with dementia, just a pound or two can often feel like a fortune, if for him the currency's pre-war value still applies.

Do not forget your humour

Difficult situations are often eased by being able to laugh at them. The dementia patient also enjoys seeing a smile on someone's face, as long as he does not feel he himself is being laughed at. One might be forgiven, for instance, for feeling sad when he wants to put some oranges under his pillow every night but, on the other hand, there is also something rather touching and amusing about it. After all, the line between happiness and sorrow is very narrow indeed. An example of this is the following brief dialogue between a nurse and a resident with dementia of a nursing home:

> *Resident to nurse*: Mummy.
> *Nurse*: I am not your mother.

Resident: If my mother is dead, would you like to be my
mother now?

(Den Tex 1990)

Remember that humour puts the brake on aggression. It is not
easy to be angry towards someone who is smiling at you. A
laughing face means, non-verbally, 'Don't hurt me – I am
not going to hurt you.' Humour always releases tension, is
liberating and gloom-dissipating.

Someone with dementia can understand the language of a
smile right up to the moment of his death. It is also one of the
first forms of communication we humans learn. A light-
hearted, not too serious approach is often the best way of
dealing with dementia.

Do not take emotional outbursts personally

Remember that emotional outbursts are often not meant
personally, but are much more expressions of helplessness. The
person with dementia knows he is losing his hold on life. This
sense of loss provokes all the same kinds of emotions we expect
to see in any mourning process: aggression, sorrow, apathy, and
so on.

When faced with anger, gloominess or suspicion (accusations), try to turn your patient's attention to something else.
Because he cannot hold on to information for any length of
time, he will soon forget what caused his negative feelings in
the first place. You will have to be very careful, however, if
the person with dementia is fully aware of his own mental
deterioration. He will see your attempts to distract him as
evidence of your not taking him seriously. Showing that you
understand his feelings can be effective here. A combination of
distraction and response to what he feels is good in all cases. If
he is unhappy because he has lost something you can suggest

that you look for it together, and then gradually steer his thoughts towards something more pleasing.

Remember that enjoyment is still possible

Do not allow yourself to be led astray by the thought: 'It doesn't make any difference what I say or do, because he will have forgotten it all within a few minutes.' If you do that, you rob yourself of the chance of making him happy now, or of giving him occasional moments of pleasure later. The person with dementia always has it in him to be happy! All that has changed is that he cannot now remember the happy moments so well as he once could. Is it not true that none of us is able to remember *all* the happy moments we have had? Furthermore, many – ranging from the wise men of the East to humanistic psychologists – regard the human capacity to concentrate fully on the here and now, without thinking about tomorrow or yesterday, as the most important sign of mental fitness.

Activities

Boredom and doing nothing the whole day long is not good for anyone, including people with on-coming dementia. On the other hand, active participation and achievement conttributes to our self-esteem, and to the feeling that we are in control of our lives. It is necessary, therefore, to devise activities which will offer enjoyment and encouragement to your patient.

It will not be easy, however, to get him working. The reason for this lies in the fact that the symptoms of his illness, such as a decreased capacity to deal with stress and noise, concentration problems, difficulty in judging what is going on around him, difficulty in following instructions, and less ability to absorb information make it well nigh impossible for him to learn anything new. It also costs him enormous effort to take the initiative in any new activity. Another problem is that, in the early stages of dementia, the patient's abilities can change from day to day.

If the following conditions are kept in mind, it should still be possible to keep someone with dementia busy and active:

- The carer should take the initiative.

- Plan activities at moments of the day when the person concerned is likely to have the most energy and is likely to be most receptive.

- Concentrate on what he is still able to do, rather than on what he is not able to do. Be realistic and bear in mind that being busy is more important than the result itself.

- Keep noise and distractions to a minimum.

- Select activities that are suitable for adults. People with dementia can feel very offended if they are asked to do things which they associate with children.

- Stop any activity immediately if there are any signs of restlessness.

- Opt preferably for activities which your patient enjoyed doing in the past.

- Offer help, but do not take the task over from him: 'let's do this together' is often the best way of creating the right atmosphere.

- Divide the activities into simple steps – this is the most effective way of working with people with dementia.

- Be careful with activities requiring scissors or needles, or other potentially dangerous implements. Keep a constant eye on this.

- Visit shops, restaurants or libraries when they are less busy. Inform personnel discreetly about the nature of the illness, especially in the case of shops and institutions you visit frequently with your patient.

- Try to introduce different activities, knowing that your patient's attention span is limited.

- Avoid activities that call for decisions. They can cause someone with dementia considerable stress.

With these conditions in mind – dependent on the phase of the illness – the following activities are often possible (taken from the Alzheimer Information Guide 1997):

Household chores: dusting; hoovering; sweeping; mopping; folding the washing; laying the table; polishing silver, brass or furniture; watering the plants and flowers.

Outdoor activities: hoeing; gardening; planting flowers; watering the flowers; weeding; mowing the lawn.

Handiwork: embroidery; stringing beads; playing 'Snap' or 'Happy Families'; making collages; transferring patterns cut on a sponge (or potato), and dipped in paint, to paper; simple sewing tasks.

Listening to music: classical music or your patient's own favourite songs; watching or participating in choral performances; attending appropriate concerts.

Reminiscing: looking through photograph albums; watching family films and videos, and viewing slides together.

Free time: window-shopping; a walk or a car ride; dancing to your patient's favourite music; attending local sports events; visiting libraries and restaurants (but not if they are busy); watching (non-violent) films; doing simple jigsaw puzzles (large pieces); physical exercises seated in a chair; listening to talking-books.

Other activities: count and sort place mats or other household articles (avoid small items which can be swallowed); 'people-watching' on the street; a relaxed cup of tea or a drink with friends or relatives in a pub or tea-room garden; adopt a household pet (if a dog or cat is not possible, perhaps a bird or fish).

8

The family
The hidden victims

Introduction

The process of drifting into dementia lasts, on average, some seven years. The illness not only affects the person in question, but those around him too; sometimes even more so than the patient himself. It is an illness that turns the lives of those closest to him completely upside down. The carers themselves differ greatly, but they nonetheless all struggle with the same worries, problems and emotions.

Common problems

All the members of the family are confronted with the pain of parting from one of their own   , someone they love. They are in the process of losing him whilst he is still alive. They have to mourn, and during that long and slow process of letting go they experience all the emotions inherent in any mourning process: denial; disbelief; rebellion; sorrow; shame; anger; loneliness; guilt; jealousy; helplessness; and so on.

The following is an account of a husband mourning his loss:

If you are living alone – and certainly if the situation is new for you – you learn to manage without the mirror, the consolidation of your personality: the feedback which can only be given by a loved one. That 'loved other' has no notion any more that she is called Carien, or Katrientje, or Kath, or Piglet; that she is married, that I am her husband; that she has children and does not know their names... That is so awful, if you add it all up; your lifetime companion has suddenly gone, the partner–lover has suddenly gone, and suddenly too the 'loved other', the one who safeguarded you against making stupid mistakes in your texts, and who was 'good' for more than 50 per cent of my/our place in the society around us, and who thereby established and secured our once so solid existence, our 'being'.

(Vergoed 1993)

A daughter describes her attempts to come to terms with her grief:

This is a slow departure. So slow that death can only come as a deliverance. You do not need to feel sad about it. You have already come to terms with that sorrow, bit by bit. Every day, another piece of the 'goodbye'. Until there is no more. It's over. You say that to yourself. Again and again. It is a kind of credo which by repeating over and over again, you ultimately come to accept. But that's not how it works, in fact. No way. It really doesn't work like that at all.

(Van den Berg 1995)

The mourning process in this case is often more difficult because, contrary to losing someone in death, there is no clear 'moment of loss' here. In working through the process, relatives of people with dementia are always running behind the facts, as it were. Just when they have accepted one particular 'loss' – such as the patient not wanting to leave the house any more – the next 'loss' appears: incontinence, for instance.

Relatives often fail to see the 'loss' for what it is: the person with dementia is still alive, after all. This, together with the lucid moments which someone with dementia can still have, can often give the wrong impression to those around him. Apart from the slow loss of a fondly loved member of the family, there is also the carer's loss of freedom. The caregiver cannot live his own life any more, because the patient's illness also takes complete hold of him, as carer, physically and mentally.

> My house has become my prison. I now have to lead his life for him, instead of leading my own. Everything centres around my husband's care needs. Even shopping is a precarious undertaking, because I don't feel happy leaving him alone. As I stand at the check-out, I am saying to myself: 'Come on, hurry up please.' My thoughts are constantly with my husband, and sometimes I offer a short prayer to God asking him to make sure that nothing happens to him while I am out of the house for a few minutes.
>
> (A wife)

Apart from the worry that something will happen to the patient, caregiving relatives also share worries about the future. One will be afraid that her health will let her down: 'Suppose I get sick – what will happen? Who will look after my husband then?' Another will be anxious about what the future will hold for someone with dementia: 'I am so afraid that my mother is deteriorating. I dare not even think about having to have her admitted to a nursing home.' Yet another is afraid that his partner will no longer recognize him.

A most common complaint voiced by relatives is that so few people show any signs of realizing what the situation actually means for the family; and some people around the patient really do not know how difficult the situation is for the caregiving relative. 'She never complains,' they say, or 'She looks so well.' Others are wise enough to say nothing, afraid as they are of being confronted by a statement like: 'Why don't you do something for Pa now and again?' Not only neighbours, but other relatives too, often have to assess the situation on the basis of very sparse information.

A daughter caring for her father put it thus:

> My brothers and sisters think I exaggerate too much. They say I take much too much out of Dad's hands, and that I see him with far too negative eyes. But they don't know just how little he is capable of now. When they visit us – for an hour, never longer than that! – I will have seen to it that he is well-dressed, and then he puts on a very good face for their benefit. I am often surprised by that. But as soon as they are out of the door, he becomes another person, in no time. I would like my brothers and sisters to see him as he really is.

Where there is a lack of understanding there is also a lack of appreciation. Many caregivers who have been caring for a relative or partner for several years notice that it was only in the beginning that appreciation of their efforts was expressed. But no longer. 'Everyone seems to take it for granted that I do all this. I am never complimented. I only ever hear any comments when, in their eyes, I am doing something wrong.'

A daughter caring for her invalid mother and her father who has dementia talked about this problem:

When my younger sister comes by, my mother can be guaranteed to say: 'How nice of you to come, you are always so busy.' But I am always busy too, because I am the one who is looking after my parents the whole day. I find Mum's comment very painful, although I know she is not really aware of what is going on. I also miss some sign of appreciation from my family. I only see my brothers at birthday parties. Perhaps they don't visit us more often because they don't quite know how to approach the situation. I find it very difficult to accept that no one ever asks how I am. The others just assume 'Oh, Carol is managing', and that's true, of course – Carol *is* coping with it all.

Almost without exception, caregivers are prone to contradictory and mixed emotions. They feel love, concern and sympathy for their partner or relative, but on the other hand they also feel anger and annoyance:

He recently found a doll's head in the street. He brought it into the kitchen, cleaned it and muttered again and again: 'What a pretty face, what a pretty face.' The whole day long. On the one hand you feel tremendous pity for him, but on the other hand...

(A partner)

Nearly all carers in this kind of situation will also have moments when they feel it's all getting out of control, and suddenly they 'explode'.

He suddenly turns round, goes into the bathroom and urinates in the sink. This infuriates me. I tell him it is dirty and messy. It is surely not necessary with three toilets in the house! As tired as I am by so much disturbed sleep, no more than a series of short naps, I turn the wrong use of the sink into an enormous drama. I lose my head completely. Justus is shocked and retreats into an impenetrable silence. He makes no response whatsoever to my verbal outburst, and without uttering a word he crawls back into bed with a 'drop dead' expression on his face. When I manage to calm down a bit, I realize why I was so incredibly angry. It was, of course, not primarily about the sink, but rather about another piece of loss of decorum.

(Prins 1997)

At a certain moment, he became totally distraught, pulling his hair out of his head. It had obviously dawned on him that the situation was not going to change. The pity you then feel is so awful, so heart-breaking, that after a period of consoling and embracing him, you just want to hit or kick someone or something. Because he is right, because you can't do anything about it, because you know you cannot bear this much longer. You think to yourself 'stop, stop, stop, please'. And sometimes you say it too.

(Wielek 1996)

Some caregivers find themselves swinging constantly between, on the one hand, the desire to look after and 'be there' for the patient and, on the other hand, the longing to be able to live their own lives, such as following a study course, a hobby, visiting friends, or taking a job.

It is not so much that I am not content to care for my mother, but it is all taking much longer than we realized at the start. Before I know it, I shall be old myself and a large part of my life will have gone. But as soon as I think about myself, my thoughts automatically turn back to my mother again. I don't seem to have found the answer yet.

(A daughter)

Most caregivers find it very difficult to ask for outside help.

I much prefer to do it alone. If you call in a stranger, you lose part of your independence and freedom. I heard from a niece who called in the help of a social nurse that the nurse – in no time – took over the whole leadership role and set about organizing everything. I don't want that.

(A partner)

Caregiving relatives often have very mixed feelings towards social workers and the like, especially in the official help application period. 'If I ask for help, others will think I can't manage, and then I would feel I had failed.' The family often experiences the arrival of the social worker or nurse as living proof of their own inability to cope with the situation. Furthermore, the 'outside carer' is often no better at the job than they. The mixed feelings lie largely in the fact that, on the one hand, the family members feel, or know, quite well that they need help, but would prefer, on the other hand, to do what is necessary without any outside help. The latter leaves them free to establish their own rhythm and routine, without having to adapt their day schedules to that of the 'stranger'.

A severely ill relative can also often constitute a seriously divisive element within both the nuclear and the extended family:

It has to be said that, strangely, in cases of dementia, constant divisions can develop between the remaining 'healthy' partner and the 'children'. I repeat here the comments I heard in the nursing home: 'This does not surprise us at all. We see it in seven or eight out of ten cases [of dementia].' And I later saw such cases at close hand which were ultimately far more disturbing than ours; intense, permanent, irreparable rifts within families, to the extent even of a member committing suicide.

(Vergoed 1993)

Arguments develop in the family around the question of who has to give the care and which form of care is the most suitable.

You know that as brothers and sisters we care about each other, that we love each other, but I still can't help feeling that there is something fundamental missing. And that's because we can't talk to each other about how Dad should be cared for.

(A daughter)

Self-care: the basis of caring for a partner or relative

Relatives involved in the care of a sick person have to address all kinds of problems, and many succeed, despite this, in sustaining that care for a long period of time. Some are also able to draw great satisfaction from their efforts, and would not want to have missed this period of their lives for anything.

It is becoming increasingly clear to me that I feel no sadness simply because she is as she is – because I know that the joy in being able to care for her springs from that sorrow. I have no more free time; I cannot leave her alone. And I know without a doubt that, if I were to find myself walking through the town on my own, I would be thinking: 'Damn it, I want Greet to be walking next to me.' And I would go back home immediately. If she goes, then it's finished for me too. I will then sink for a time into the memories of her, and feel extreme gratitude for everything we shared together, without understanding what I had done to deserve it. Precisely because she is as she is now, I see how happy I am.

(Ruigrok 1994)

One trap you can fall into as a carer is to subordinate your own health and well-being to that of your partner or relative with dementia. This is a real pitfall, because the caring task runs more smoothly and gives greater satisfaction if you give due regard to your own physical and mental health. The better you care for your own needs, the better you can care for the other. If you are relaxed and feel rested you will be more successful in creating the relaxed and untroubled atmosphere your patient needs.

That is easily said, of course, but how do you actually do it? Here are a few tips:

- Try to accustom your partner, or relative with dementia, to the fact that several people will be involved in his care. In this way, you will prevent him thinking that you are the only person who can help him (see Clinging behaviour in Chapter 6).

- Bear in mind that organizing the necessary care may perhaps cost you more time and energy than you initially might seem to get back from it. In the long term, however, you will be able to harvest the fruits and it will help you to prevent yourself from becoming isolated from the world around you.

- Don't be over-caring. Your patient needs to be mobile and take exercise. Leave the room, or turn your head away, if you feel yourself getting impatient at the slowness of your patient's pace. If you think he is having difficulties with something, don't take it over from him. Pity is a poor adviser.

- Make time occasionally to reflect on your own feelings. It often helps too to talk to a trusted friend about how you feel.

- Try to take a realistic look at your emotions, such as guilt, shame and jealousy. Don't bottle them up. That is dangerous: both for yourself, and for those around you. If you prefer not to talk about your feelings, it can help to put them down on paper, in a diary for instance. It also helps to try to turn negative feelings into positive actions: tidy a cupboard, do some cleaning, take a walk or a bike-ride, give someone a call, etc.

- Be aware of the fact that it becomes even more difficult to create more space for yourself if you have already completely submerged yourself for a long time in the caring needs of your patient. If you try to break this pattern, nervousness and feelings of guilt are perfectly normal. The best way to break a set pattern concentrated solely on care is to take the gradual road. You might start, for instance, by taking one free afternoon a fortnight to do some personal shopping, or to work on a favourite hobby elsewhere.

- Allow yourself 'one treat' a day, so that you always have something to look forward to. Examples: telephone your (grand)children every day; play the piano, or listen to favourite music, for half an hour; read a magazine or book; go for a good walk; potter about in the garden.

- If another problem arises, think about how you might be able to get some extra help. Don't assume that you will have to solve it on your own. Everyone is different, and everyone experiences a situation differently. What one will view quite calmly, another will find very irritating. Never blame yourself for your emotions.

- Remember that we all make mistakes and fall short from time to time. Caring for a partner, relative or friend who has dementia is so demanding that no one could possibly do it perfectly all the time. And nor can you.

- Remember that few people can read another's thoughts. Try to say as clearly as possible what you think and feel; and realize that many 'outsiders' have an incorrect picture of the situation. They base their judgement on what they see at any given moment. Do not expect them to include in their judgement of that moment the (long) period that preceded it, unless of course you have already made it as clear as possible.

- Your own needs and wishes can often clash with those of the person for whom you are caring. Try not to be too self-effacing, and try not to become a martyr or a saint. 'Give and take' is the motto or, in other words, 'share the misery fairly'. In the long term, this is by far the best strategy for both of you.

- Avoid becoming isolated. If it proves impossible to visit other people, then invite them to come to you. Explain honestly why you cannot go to them. Don't worry about what they think or say about you, about your patient, or about your house. What is important is that you have company around you. (Remember too that it is also in the interests of your patient to maintain contact with the world 'outside': it enriches his life too.)

- Set priorities all the time. Make lists of what is most important for you, and try as much as possible to stick to them. Do the things that must be done on that day, followed at your leisure by the other less urgent chores.

- Tell your relatives and friends what you know about dementia. Tell them what dementia does to someone's memory, mind and personality, and how they themselves can best communicate with the person with dementia during their visits. This helps to prevent uncomfortable situations which may lead to would-be visitors staying away. Visitors then have a better idea of how to approach your patient. And remember that it is often men who have the most difficulty in dealing with dementia.

- Caring for another is not purely a litany of strife and misery. On the contrary, it is also possible to derive pleasure and satisfaction from it, as many carers will testify. Try to concentrate on the positive sides of giving care. Just as it is important to talk with others about your negative feelings, so too is it worthwhile allowing others to share in your more optimistic feelings, in the pleasing moments, and in the satisfaction you get from caring for your partner or relative. Do not worry about being accused of bragging or self-satisfaction, but think more in terms of 'shared pleasure is double pleasure'.

- Try not to fret about the other all the time. If he was not suffering from dementia, you probably wouldn't be fretting at all, and your concern and anxiousness will not help him to feel any better.

- It is a misconception to think that there is always a perfect solution to every problem; there are usually several possible solutions to every problem. Let your imagination get to work, and don't allow yourself to be put off by obstacles or objections. Commit possible solutions to paper; pick out the two or three possibilities you think are most appropriate, and then list the pros and cons. You can then make the final choice, and see that in most cases there is indeed a suitable way out of the problem.

- Read these tips regularly. Do not try to take all the advice 'on board' in one go, but choose one (each time) and make a serious attempt to apply it.

9

Feelings of guilt

Introduction

Nearly everyone who is confronted with dementia in the family will, sooner or later, be troubled by feelings of guilt. For many, these feelings of guilt often have the effect of pushing all their other emotions into the background, and this may last for many years. Feelings of guilt can play a central role in how relatives view the situation, hence there being a separate chapter devoted to this aspect. We will look, first of all, at the sources of guilt, and then at their meaning and at what lies behind them. Finally, we will offer a few suggestions on how to deal with such emotions.

Guilt after hearing the diagnosis

As soon as family members are informed that the strange behaviour exhibited by their relative is caused by dementia, they struggle with the realization that they probably failed, and misunderstood, him on many occasions in the past. They deeply regret the arguments, the scoldings and the rows, and they know now that their demands were unrealistic; 'he wouldn't...' or 'he didn't really try...' was, in fact, 'he couldn't...'.

Relatives often show deep remorse for having allowed a period to pass in which they could have had much more pleasure together. Or they are sorry that they did not actually ask the questions they wanted to have answered. Questions, for instance, about decisions the father, mother, uncle or aunt who have dementia had made in the past.

Some are desperate to know whether something they did, or did not do, caused or worsened the illness. In the stories that relatives tell us, we regularly see their regret at not having been aware of the fact that dementia was playing a role in the situation, that they did not know what the effects of the illness were, or what are the most important rules for interacting effectively with dementia patients. Sometimes they point the finger of suspicion at the patient's general practitioner or the treating specialist, but equally often the accusation veils their own struggle with self-blame: 'I should have asked for information earlier', or 'I should not have turned a deaf ear to what others were telling me.'

Relatives who are told by others that they always did the best they could, and that that is the only thing that counts, continue to feel guilty nonetheless. And even when they know that knowledge alone is no guarantee that things will ever go smoothly and without problems, they are still nagged by a troubled conscience. They are not even helped by being told that professional carers too – despite all their knowledge and experience – can still 'go wrong' when dementia affects someone in their own families.

> I worked as a nurse for many years caring for old people, and I had seen many cases of dementia. That all went perfectly well until I noticed that my mother was also starting to show signs of dementia. I could not, and would not, accept it. My mum – no, that was not possible. Oh, the struggle I put up then! I had so much pity for this

woman. She was so good and so honest! I was so angry that my mother would have to endure this. At the start of dementia, you blame everything and everyone. And when you think you are doing all the right things, it becomes apparent that you are doing all the wrong things. I couldn't cope with it.

(A daughter)

It is never enough

Once family members know that their relative is suffering from dementia, have accepted the diagnosis, and are determined to put great efforts into supporting the patient and giving him the care he needs, feelings of guilt even then do not go away. It seems, in fact, that they often become even more intense. Relatives often blame themselves for being insufficiently tactful, loving and calm, for not being able to bring the patient out of his isolation, and for not being able to relieve his suffering, etc. In short, they blame themselves for not doing enough, or for not giving sufficient care.

I think this is the hardest lesson about Alzheimer's disease for a caregiver: you can never do enough to make a difference in the course of the disease. Hard because what we feel anyway is that we have never done enough. We blame ourselves. We always find ourselves deficient in devotion. Did you visit once a week? You might have visited twice. Oh, you visited daily? But perhaps he would have done better if you'd kept him at home. In the end all those judgements, those self-judgements, are pointless. The disease is inexorable, cruel. It scoffs at everything.

Still, still we look to ourselves to have made a difference. We remember everything we didn't do. This

gets played out in painful ways in families too, when one
person takes on the caregiving responsibility. Sometimes I
wished my siblings would do more – as though that
would have made any difference! Just as, when my father
was in Denver and my sister had responsibility for him,
she felt we others didn't do enough. It is costly,
emotionally, to watch someone move inevitably, step by
step, into a dementing illness, and it's hard not to want to
blame someone – ourselves most of all. But it's useless.

(Miller 2003)

You might expect relatives to be more troubled by feelings of
guilt if they do less for the person with dementia and that, by
the same token, feelings of guilt will be less intense in those
who do more for the patient. The opposite is more likely to be
true, however. Those providing the bulk of the care, in fact,
tend to suffer the most severe feelings of guilt. Many of these
caregiving relatives go to the utmost limits of what can
reasonably be expected of them in their care of the partner or
relative with dementia, and some even go beyond those limits.
Despite their amazing and noble efforts, they feel permanently
guilty. Feelings of guilt are quite separate, therefore, from the
degree of care given. In other words, feelings of guilt pervade
even when the carer is doing everything he or she possibly can.

Feelings of guilt in those who provide most of the care
stem from the demands made on them from three or four sides.
First, there are the demands the caregivers place on themselves.
Not a few of them, for instance, impose the impossible demand
on themselves to satisfy all the patient's physical and mental
needs in every way, every day, that he must not suffer, and that
he must not be unhappy. 'You want to see your father happy.
And if he is not, then that is very difficult to cope with.' And
when this is indeed the case, the carer will see it as his/her own
failure.

Second, the patient demands a great deal of the caregiver. The appeal the person with dementia makes on his carer can change from day to day, and sometimes from hour to hour: 'At one moment he can do everything, and a few minutes, or an hour later, he can do nothing, and he can then put on a very pathetic face indeed. And at moments like that, I want to slap him.'

Third, there is the immediate family, the children for instance, who also have their own expectations: 'Mum, other mothers help their children with homework, but you spend every evening with Granny.'

And finally, there are the carer's own longings and desires, and they cannot be ignored forever: 'I like painting; no, no Rembrandt-like masterpieces – I simply enjoy brushing a layer of paint onto doors or fences. My hands just itch sometimes to hold a paint-brush and get to work, but the last time I did that was some two years ago.'

There are professionals, too, who expect things of the relatives. It is not surprising, therefore, that family members can feel very trapped in this web of demanding networks, pulling at them from all sides. It is not possible to please everyone all the time, and this is often yet another reason for carers to feel guilty. The more they do for the person at the centre of it all, the less they can do for others.

Admission to a nursing home

Dad rings me and says in an expressionless voice: 'She can go to the nursing home tomorrow.' Tomorrow? But that's Kirsten's birthday.

I go. I realise in the car that the house I am driving to will, from today onwards, never be the same. The house I grew up in, the house I know every inch of. The house where Mum lives. Lived.

Mum is standing in the middle of the room, lost.

'She wants to take her sewing box with her,' Dad says despairingly.

'Mum, shall I look after your sewing box for you?' I ask.

She agrees. She walks with us to the car, not understanding where she is going. Not realising that it will be permanent. Because we have never dared to take her back, for fear that she would recognize her house. We later leave the nursing home, without exchanging any words. Vague tears roll over the cheeks of that well-built man who has no choice but to leave his wife in the nursing home. In my pocket, I hold the labels I have to sew into my mother's clothes firmly in my fist.

We drive to my house, where there are paper chains and visitors. I quickly push a gift into Dad's hand which he then presents to his youngest granddaughter.

(Van den Berg 1995)

In many cases, there comes a moment when the family can no longer provide the care needed, and the only option open to them then is to prepare the way for admission to a nursing home. It is a myth to imagine that people in the early stages of dementia in this country are all too easily 'dumped' in a nursing home. Families usually wait until the situation is almost completely untenable, and they themselves are on the brink of exhaustion and despair, before they face up to the prospect of nursing home care for their relative with dementia. Sometimes the die is only cast after the family's general practitioner has exerted the necessary pressure on the caring partner or the children.

These caregivers are often troubled by the same feelings as parents of a mentally handicapped child confronting the painful realization that the care of their beloved child will soon be handed over to specialized staff in a specialized home. Sending 'a vulnerable, defenceless being' away from his home and family is, in their view, 'an inhuman act'. Is the relative with dementia not a 'defenceless being' too? For a carer-daughter, her mother or father can often become an 'adopted child'. Many women who have cared for one or both of their parents over a long period of time admit that they would never be able to accept a similar sacrifice from their own children. They would have no hesitation in accepting admission to a nursing home. It is only with the utmost effort that they are able to surmount the 'guilt barrier' in order to prepare the way for mother or father to be admitted to a nursing home. And they often look back on such a step as 'being the most difficult decision of my life'.

> My brother always refers to January 3rd 1994 as the worst day of his life. At half past one that afternoon, he brings Dad to the 'Hof', a home for ageing dementia patients. Someone had to take Dad there, and my brother was the first to step forward when volunteers were asked for. I do not envy him: leaving Dad there must have felt like committing high treason.
>
> We all know that the 'Hof' means a 'life sentence'. And we also know that Dad is well aware of these things, even though that realization may only be occasional and brief. One second is long enough for profound sorrow.
>
> (Hilhorst 1999)

Many are haunted by the question of whether or not it was a good decision to have their parent admitted to a nursing home.

The moment the family is informed that the nursing home is now able to accept the patient, relatives will often want to go back on their decision, or delay admission for a while. Consciously, or subconsciously, there is always the hope that death will quickly intervene and thus make the question of admission totally superfluous. Once again, thoughts like these can provoke severe feelings of guilt.

Once admission to the nursing home has become reality, however, the feelings of guilt rise to the surface again for many. Although, on the one hand, family members feel a sense of relief, there is also the nagging thought: 'If only we had been able to keep Ma or Pa at home longer.' It is a thought that arises most often several weeks later, when the relatives have been able to catch their breath and recharge their batteries. The intensity of these feelings ebbs away in the course of time, however. The sharpest aspects of the emotion lessen in time, especially as the family see that their relative with dementia has settled well into the nursing home. For many, however, the 'wound' caused by the guilt nags on for many years, and every visit can re-open that wound. The sight of father or mother sitting at a table, lonely amongst all the other people with dementia – staring into nothing, dozing, muttering, talking loudly to themselves, screaming, dribbling food or drink down themselves – is something very difficult to accept. As someone once said: 'Nothing is more distressing than seeing the suffering of someone one loves and not being able to help. Seeing a loved one suffer is worse than having to suffer oneself.'

Being enthusiastically welcomed by the relative with dementia – a moment of true recognition shining on his face – is not only a happy moment for those closest to him, but it can also disturb their consciences again. The most painful moment is having to leave him again, the wave at the door ever-reminiscent of the real moment of parting: the day he was admitted to the nursing home. Visits that could not be made – a schedule of daily visits is too demanding for the former principal carer, perhaps, or the distance is too great, or the carer herself is not well and has to see the doctor, and so on – can also provoke feelings of guilt. Relatives who, for all kinds of reasons, cannot visit the patient might be so conscience-stricken that they cannot resist asking the returning visitor: 'Did he ask about me?' Some of the statements made by the patient with dementia must almost certainly also add fuel to the fire of a burning conscience when, for instance, they say something like: 'Are you going to take me home with you today?', or 'It's just like a prison in here.'

It would not be an exaggeration to say that for very many family members who felt they had no choice but to hand over the care of their well-loved relative with dementia to a nursing home, hardly a day, and sometimes not even an hour, goes by without their feeling uneasy and unhappy about it. Research has shown that the ex-carers of relatives admitted to a nursing home experience no less stress after admission than they did before it.

The nature of the psychological burden, however, is very different. Caring turns into worrying. In practically every talk carers have with someone they trust, the discussion turns almost inevitably to the subject of the 'nursing home'. They *have* to talk about it, otherwise they will have no peace of mind, although, in practice, talking about it brings no definite end to their pangs of conscience. There is an old saying that says: time heals all wounds; sadly, however, this kind of guilt feeling has all the appearances of being permanent, and can even persist long after the patient has died.

The psychological meaning

Where do feelings of guilt come from? Modern-day psychology regards feelings as 'action-tendencies': feelings and emotions spur us into action. Love stimulates us to want to be as close as we possibly can to the one we love. Anger urges us to do something to the other, to retaliate. Feelings of guilt stimulate us to nullify our past faults and shortcomings – and we do this via a backward movement. As soon as we discover that we can never bring the past into the present, our feelings of guilt then spur us on to bear the pain and do penance. And we do that by means of self-accusation – the magical instrument we use to 'settle the accounts' of the past.

Feelings of guilt often take little, or no, account of what is reasonable. They whisper to us that we could always have done *more*. Just as yearning is always larger than ourselves – after every success we always want more, another rung higher on the ladder – the horizon of our feeling of guilt moves simultaneously with every effort and with every self-sacrificing step we take. The reason for this is that feelings of guilt have an important psychological purpose. In cultures in which everything is believed to be pre-destined, as in India for instance, feelings of guilt do not exist. We Westerners, however, believe strongly that our own efforts really do make a difference. Without feelings of guilt, life would be one big game of chance, including our contracting – or not contracting – a fatal illness, our own capacities, the moment of admission to a nursing home, and so forth. We *cannot* believe that, and we do not *want* to believe it. Behind every feeling of guilt there is an almost child-like feeling of power, the thought that there is a tiny piece of God in all of us. The psychological purpose of guilt, therefore, is that it drives us to control our own lives; and because we need to do this so badly, feelings of guilt can be very persistent indeed.

Past guilt – paying off the debt

Feelings of guilt not only torment the partner of someone with dementia – the children of that union are also plagued by much the same emotions, even though they, unlike the partner at the time of the marriage, never vowed to care for either parent in sickness and in health, for better or for worse.

The American psychologist Brody (1984) explains the guilt feelings of children in the following terms: in the first phase of our lives, we receive from our young parents all the care and devotion appropriate to our state of total dependence. During this period, the idea develops deep in our subconscious that we have a moral duty to repay this debt if, and when, our parents themselves become dependent on the care of others. It is impossible, however, to pay off this moral debt by giving the same total care as we received in our childhood. The roles of parents and children can never be completely reversed. It is this inescapability – the difference that remains in our minds – which leads to feelings of guilt. Women usually battle more often with feelings of guilt than men. The most plausible explanation for this is that women relate their self-esteem and their self-assurance primarily to their capacity to be caring. If there is a risk of the care for the person in need falling short, women often blame themselves: 'I have failed; I have failed as a woman.'

Men, on the other hand, derive their self-respect not so much from providing care, but more often from their career roles outside the home. Care problems thus tend far less often to turn into personal dramas for them.

Handling feelings of guilt

How should we handle feelings of guilt? First, it can help enormously to know that these feelings of guilt are perfectly normal. This also explains why an entire chapter of this book has been devoted to the subject.

The best coping strategy for feelings of guilt, therefore, is to acknowledge them: 'Yes, I feel guilty.' If we accept troublesome emotions for what they are, we have a better chance of being able to contain them. The more we resist them, the more powerful they become. We could compare them to a large dog: the more we show our fear and the more we try to chase him off, the more he growls and the more dangerous he becomes.

Finally, it also helps to talk about our feelings. We take a step forward every time we talk to someone about them. The pain will decrease on each subsequent occasion – bit by bit, therefore, the deep, dark, well of guilt will lessen. It is best to talk about feelings of guilt with people who understand the situation, such as those who are, or have been, in more or less 'the same boat'.

> And we talk with other families, because relatives of the residents seek each other out in the nursing home. We are all part of it. We understand each other. People who have had to leave their partners here cling to each other for support and confirmation. It is comforting to know that one's feelings are not abnormal. He feels the same, and so does she. Because we all feel guilty.
>
> 'I fret such a lot – could I not have coped for a bit longer?' one lady says hesitatingly.
>
> My father nods.
>
> 'That fall she had – that would never have happened if she had been under my care at home,' he says sadly.
>
> And another says with some reluctance: 'He is deteriorating so fast here. When he was still at home, I could keep him in touch with the world a bit.'
>
> 'Sometimes I think, I'll take him home with me...'

Guilt continues to haunt our minds. If we see something we are not happy about in the home, we do not complain to the nursing staff. They, after all, have taken over the task we failed to complete. We can only say that – in so many words – to each other.

We confirm each other. Indeed, there is no other way. It is really better as it is. We hear others saying things we have known for a long time.

We cannot do it. Caring, watching, guarding for 24 hours a day. A job, a family, children... We all have a viable excuse. And yet... The guilt remains. We carry it with us the whole way – from the moment of admission to the home, right to the end. I have let her down. That's how it feels, anyway.

(Van den Berg 1995)

Experience with discussion groups comprising partners and relatives of people with dementia has shown that participants in such groups are most likely to learn more about the phenomenon of dementia from them, and about the ways relatives can best approach and help the person directly concerned. They also learn how best to deal with their own emotions by exchanging ideas and experiences with others. Recognizing the feelings of others in the same, or similar, situation often results in relatives being able to openly acknowledge how they feel deep inside, and often in coming closer also to acceptance.

A priest or church minister is another possible source of welcome solace. Feelings of guilt function, as we have already seen, as a kind of act of penance: we feel we have to suffer. A religious ritual such as confession – familiar to Roman Catholics – can, in certain cases, have a very healing effect. The ritual washes the soul clean of the black stain of guilt, so that the person concerned feels able once again to stand in front of his/her own moral mirror.

References

Alzheimer-informatiegids [Alzheimer Information Guide] (1997) 'Internationale Stichting Alzheimer Onderzoek.' Hoofddorp: ISAO.

Avontroodt, Y. (2002) 'Er groeit een nieuwe persoonlijkheid.' [A new personality is developing here.] In A. van Keymeulen (ed) *Het dementiecafé*. [The dementia coffee house.] Berchem: Epo.

Bayley, J. (1999) *Elegy for Iris*. New York: St Martin's Press.

Bayley, J. (2000) *Iris and her friends. A memoir of memory and desire*. New York: W.W. Norton & Company.

Berg, M. van den (1995) *Ze is de vioolmuziek vergeten*. [She has forgotten the violin music.] Den Bosch: Van Reemst.

Bernlef, J. (1988) *Out of mind*. London: Faber and Faber.

Braak, H. and Braak, E. (1996) 'Development of Alzheimer related neurofibrilary changes in the neocortex inversaly recaptulates cortical myelogenesis.' *Acta Neuropathogical 92*, 197–201.

Brody, E.M. (1984) 'Parent care as a normative family stress.' *The Gerontologist 25*, 19–29.

Buijssen, H. and Razenberg, I. (1991) *Dementie. Een praktische handreiking voor de omgang met Alzheimer patiënten*. [Dementia. A caregiver's guide.] Meppel: Boom.

Buñuel, L. (2003) *My last sigh*. Mineapolis: University of Minnesota Press. Translated by Abigail Israel.

Cioni, G., Biagioni, E. and Cipollini, C. (1992) 'Brain before cognition: EEG maturation in preterm infants.' In I. Kostovic, S. Knezevic, H.M. Wisnieski and G.J. Spillich (eds) *Neurodevelopment, aging and cognition*. Boston: Birkhäuser.

Delft, I.H. van (1993) *We komen niet meer waar we geweest zijn. Demente bejaarden aan het woord*. [We no longer go where we have been before.] Baarn: Anthos.

Duijnstee, M. (1996) *Het verhaal achter de feiten. Over de belasting van dementerende familieleden*. [The story behind the facts. About the stress of caring for victims of dementia.] Thesis. Baarn: HBuitgevers.

Franssen, E.H., Souren, L.E.M., Torossian, C.L. and Reisberg, B. (1997) 'Utility of the developmental reflexes in the differential diagnosis and prognosis of incontinence in Alzheimer's disease.' *Journal of Geriatric Psychiatry and Neurology 10*, 22–28.

Grant, L. (1998) *Remind me who I am again*. London: Granta Books.

Hilhorst, M. (1999) *De vader, de moeder & de tijd.* [The father, the mother and the time.] Amsterdam: Meulenhoff.

Ignatieff, M. (1993) *Scar Tissue.* London: Chattoo & Windus.

Kooy, C. van der (2003) *Gewoon lief zijn?* [Just being nice?] Thesis. Utrecht: Lemma.

Lange, J. de (2004) *Omgaan met dementie.* [Dealing with dementia.] Thesis. Utrecht: Trimbos-instituut.

Luria, A.R. (1992) *The man with a shattered world.* Cambridge, MA: Harvard University Press. Translated by Lynn Solotoroff.

Mahy, M. (1987) *Memory.* London: Collins Flamingo.

Marquez, G. (1988) *Love in the time of cholera.* New York: Alfred A. Knopf.

Miller, S. (2003) *The story of my father.* New York: Alfred A. Knopf.

Pols, J. (1992) 'Dementie, taal en teken. Een semiotisch onderzoek bij dementerende ouderen.' [Dementia, language and sign. A semiotic study of elderly people with dementia.] *MGV 7/8,* 809–826.

Prins, S. (1997) *Dubbel verlies.* [Double loss.] Utrecht: Kosmos.

Reisberg, B. (1986) 'Dementia. A systematic approach to identifying reversible causes.' *Geriatrics 41,* 30–46.

Reisberg, B., Ferris, S.H. and Franssen, E. (1986) 'Functional degenerative stages in dementia of the Alzheimer's type appear to reverse normal human development.' In C. Shagass, R. Josiassen, W.H. Bridger, K. Weiss, D. Stoff and G.M. Simpson (eds) *Biological psychiatry.* New York: Elsevier Science.

Ruigrok, H. (1994) 'Alles is goed gekomen. Dolf Brouwers en de zin van het bestaan.' [Everything has turned out fine. Dolf Brouwers and the meaning of being.] *Nieuwe Revu 8,* 52–54.

Sclan, S.G., Foster, J.R., Reisberg, B., Franssen, E. and Welkowitz, J. (1990) 'Application of Piagetan measures of cognitive in severe Alzheimer's disease.' *Psychiatric Journal of the University of Ottawa 15,* 221–226.

Tex, U. den (1990) 'Thuis is ergens anders en nergens meer te vinden.' [Home is somewhere else and nowhere to be found.] *Vrij Nederland 17,* 6–19.

Verdult, R. (1993) *Dement worden. Een kinderetijd in beeld.* [Developing dementia.] Baarn: HBuitgevers.

Vergoed, C. (1993) 'Carien.' *Het drama van dementie.* [Carien. The tragedy of dementia.] Abcoude: Uniepers.

Voskuil, J.J. (1999) *De moeder van Nicolien.* [The mother of Nicolien.] Amsterdam: G.A. van Oorschot.

Wielek, W. (1996) 'Meegesleurd in de hel van een Alzheimerpatiënt.' [Dragged into the world of an Alzheimer patient.] *Opzij,* 40–42.

Zomeren, K. van (1987) *Een jaar in scherven.* [A year in pieces.] Amsterdam: De Arbeiderspers.

Zomeren, K. van (2001) *De man van de Middenweg.* [The man of the middle of the road.] Amsterdam: De Arbeiderspers.

Subject index

Author index